An American Crisis

The Growing Absence of Black Men in Medicine and Science

PROCEEDINGS OF A JOINT WORKSHOP

Cato T. Laurencin, M.D., Ph.D., *Rapporteur*

Board on Population Health and Public Health Practice

Health and Medicine Division

The National Academies of
SCIENCES · ENGINEERING · MEDICINE

THE NATIONAL ACADEMIES PRESS
Washington, DC
www.nap.edu

THE NATIONAL ACADEMIES PRESS 500 Fifth Street, NW Washington, DC 20001

This activity was supported by the Aetna Foundation (Contract 10003873), Burroughs Wellcome Fund (Contract 10003742), W. Montague Cobb/NMA Health Institute (unnumbered), The Kavli Foundation (10003589), National Academy of Medicine (unnumbered), National Institutes of Health (unnumbered), and the Robert Wood Johnson Foundation (Contract 10003809). Any opinions, findings, conclusions, or recommendations expressed in this publication do not necessarily reflect the views of any organization or agency that provided support for the project.

International Standard Book Number-13: 978-0-309-47690-4
International Standard Book Number-10: 0-309-47690-9
Digital Object Identifier: https://doi.org/10.17226/25130

Additional copies of this publication are available for sale from the National Academies Press, 500 Fifth Street, NW, Keck 360, Washington, DC 20001; (800) 624-6242 or (202) 334-3313; http://www.nap.edu.

Printed in the United States of America

Suggested citation: National Academies of Sciences, Engineering, and Medicine. 2018. *An American crisis: The growing absence of Black men in medicine and science: Proceedings of a joint workshop between the National Academies of Sciences, Engineering, and Medicine and the W. Montague Cobb/NMA Health Institute*. Washington, DC: The National Academies Press. doi: https://doi.org/10.17226/25130.

The National Academies of

SCIENCES • ENGINEERING • MEDICINE

The **National Academy of Sciences** was established in 1863 by an Act of Congress, signed by President Lincoln, as a private, nongovernmental institution to advise the nation on issues related to science and technology. Members are elected by their peers for outstanding contributions to research. Dr. Marcia McNutt is president.

The **National Academy of Engineering** was established in 1964 under the charter of the National Academy of Sciences to bring the practices of engineering to advising the nation. Members are elected by their peers for extraordinary contributions to engineering. Dr. C. D. Mote, Jr., is president.

The **National Academy of Medicine** (formerly the Institute of Medicine) was established in 1970 under the charter of the National Academy of Sciences to advise the nation on medical and health issues. Members are elected by their peers for distinguished contributions to medicine and health. Dr. Victor J. Dzau is president.

The three Academies work together as the **National Academies of Sciences, Engineering, and Medicine** to provide independent, objective analysis and advice to the nation and conduct other activities to solve complex problems and inform public policy decisions. The National Academies also encourage education and research, recognize outstanding contributions to knowledge, and increase public understanding in matters of science, engineering, and medicine.

Learn more about the National Academies of Sciences, Engineering, and Medicine at **www.nationalacademies.org**.

Consensus Study Reports published by the National Academies of Sciences, Engineering, and Medicine document the evidence-based consensus on the study's statement of task by an authoring committee of experts. Reports typically include findings, conclusions, and recommendations based on information gathered by the committee and the committee's deliberations. Each report has been subjected to a rigorous and independent peer-review process and it represents the position of the National Academies on the statement of task.

Proceedings published by the National Academies of Sciences, Engineering, and Medicine chronicle the presentations and discussions at a workshop, symposium, or other event convened by the National Academies. The statements and opinions contained in proceedings are those of the participants and are not endorsed by other participants, the planning committee, or the National Academies.

For information about other products and activities of the National Academies, please visit www.nationalacademies.org/about/whatwedo.

PLANNING COMMITTEE ON INCREASING AFRICAN AMERICAN MALES IN THE MEDICAL PROFESSION[1]

CATO T. LAURENCIN (*Chair*), University of Connecticut
KENDALL CAMPBELL, East Carolina University Brody School of Medicine
THEODORE J. CORBIN, Drexel University College of Medicine
GEORGE C. HILL, Vanderbilt University
RANDALL C. MORGAN, JR., W. Montague Cobb/NMA Health Institute
ELIZABETH OFILI, Morehouse School of Medicine
VIVIAN PINN, National Institutes of Health (*retired*)

Health and Medicine Division Staff

N. RENEE GETHERS, Project Director (*from January 2018*)
LESLIE Y. KWAN, Associate Program Officer (*from March 2018*)
HOPE HARE, Administrative Assistant
ROSE MARIE MARTINEZ, Project Director (*until January 2018*), Senior Board Director, Board on Population Health and Public Health Practice

[1] The National Academies of Sciences, Engineering, and Medicine's planning committees are solely responsible for organizing the workshop, identifying topics, and choosing speakers. The responsibility for the published Proceedings of a Joint Workshop rests with the workshop rapporteur and the institution.

Reviewers

This Proceedings of a Joint Workshop was reviewed in draft form by individuals chosen for their diverse perspectives and technical expertise. The purpose of this independent review is to provide candid and critical comments that will assist the National Academies of Sciences, Engineering, and Medicine in making each published proceedings as sound as possible and to ensure that it meets the institutional standards for quality, objectivity, evidence, and responsiveness to the charge. The review comments and draft manuscript remain confidential to protect the integrity of the process.

We thank the following individuals for their review of this proceedings:

L. D. BRITT, Eastern Virginia Medical School
EVE J. HIGGINBOTHAM, University of Pennsylvania
FAITH MITCHELL, Grantmakers In Health
VALERIE MONTGOMERY RICE, Morehouse School of Medicine
ALVIN POUSSAINT, Harvard Medical School
JOHN A. RICH, Drexel University School of Public Health
DARLA THOMPSON, The George Washington University

Although the reviewers listed above provided many constructive comments and suggestions, they were not asked to endorse the content of the proceedings nor did they see the final draft before its release. The review of this proceedings was overseen by **CARMEN R. GREEN,**

University of Michigan. She was responsible for making certain that an independent examination of this proceedings was carried out in accordance with standards of the National Academies and that all review comments were carefully considered. Responsibility for the final content rests entirely with the rapporteur and the National Academies.

Contents

Boxes and Figures

BOXES

FIGURES

Acronyms and Abbreviations

AAMC	Association of American Medical Colleges
AHEC	Area Health Education Center
AOA	American Osteopathic Association
APA	American Psychological Association
BHW	Bureau of Health Workforce
BUILD	Building Infrastructure Leading to Diversity initiative
CHC	community health center
DO	Doctor of Osteopathic Medicine
FDA	Food and Drug Administration
GRE	Graduate Record Examinations
HBCU	Historically Black Colleges and Universities
HCOP	Health Careers Opportunity Program
HHS	U.S. Department of Health and Human Services
HPPI	Health Professions Partnership Initiative
HRSA	Health Resources and Services Administration
LCME	Liaison Committee on Medical Education

MATC	Milwaukee Area Technical College
MCAT	Medical College Admission Test
MD	Doctor of Medicine
NAM	National Academy of Medicine
NCAA	National Collegiate Athletic Association
NHSC	National Health Service Corps
NIH	National Institutes of Health
NMA	National Medical Association
NMF	National Medical Fellowships
NSF	National Science Foundation
SES	socioeconomic status
STEM	science, technology, engineering, and mathematics
UConn	University of Connecticut
UMBC	University of Maryland, Baltimore County
UNC	University of North Carolina
UT	University of Texas
VUSM	Vanderbilt University School of Medicine

1

Introduction[1]

Black men are increasingly underrepresented in medical schools and in the medical profession. As Louis Sullivan, M.D.,[2] noted in his keynote speech, although Black[3] Americans constitute 13 percent of the U.S. population, they make up less than 7 percent of medical students and less than 3 percent of practicing physicians.[4] Moreover, according to the Association of American Medical Colleges 2014 report *Altering the Course: Black Males in Medicine*, although the proportion of Black students in medical schools has increased in the past several decades, the gains are entirely attributable to advances among Black women. By contrast, in the same period, the number of Black men in medical schools *decreased*. For example, only 515 Black or African American men matriculated to medical school in 2014 compared with 542 in 1978. Furthermore, whereas the numbers of male and female medical students are approximately equal for most racial and

[1] The planning committee's role was limited to planning the workshop, and the Proceedings of a Joint Workshop was prepared by the workshop rapporteur as a factual summary of what occurred at the workshop. Statements, recommendations, and opinions expressed are those of individual presenters and participants, and are not necessarily endorsed or verified by the National Academies of Sciences, Engineering, and Medicine, and they should not be construed as reflecting any group consensus.

[2] Sullivan is chairman and chief executive officer of The Sullivan Alliance to Transform the Health Professions and president emeritus of the Morehouse School of Medicine.

[3] The planning committee prefers the use of the term *Black*. However, throughout the proceedings, the terminology used reflects the language used by individual participants or in original sources.

[4] See Chapter 2 for discussion of Sullivan's keynote address.

ethnic groups, there are substantially more Black female medical students than Black men. Of note, this contrasts with gains in representation among other racial and ethnic minorities in medicine.[5] Despite these advances, many minority groups remain underrepresented in medicine and science. This problem is particularly acute among Black men.

Victor Dzau, M.D., president of the National Academy of Medicine (NAM), remarked that a diverse workforce is a key attribute of quality health care.[6] As he and Sullivan both remarked, research suggests that a diverse workforce may help to advance cultural competency and increase access to high-quality health care, especially for underserved populations. Conversely, lack of diversity in the health workforce threatens health care quality and access and contributes to health disparities. In this way, the growing absence of Black men in medicine is especially troubling, because their absence in medicine may have adverse consequences for health care access, quality, and outcomes among Black Americans and Americans overall.

A concerted initiative to explore ideas, especially new ideas, to effectively address the issues surrounding the lack of Black men in medicine began with the W. Montague Cobb/NMA Health Institute (Cobb Institute), its founding chair of the board, Cato T. Laurencin, M.D., Ph.D.,[7] and the Connecticut Legislative Black and Puerto Rican Caucus of the Connecticut General Assembly. At the same time, Laurencin and Marsha Murray, M.S.,[8] published "An American Crisis: The Lack of Black Men in Medicine" in the *Journal of Racial and Ethnic Health Disparities*, a publication of the Cobb Institute. The article, which the NAM reprinted as a discussion paper, called for, among many things, a national dialogue on the subject of Black men in medicine.[9]

To better understand the factors that contribute to the low participation of Black men in the medical profession, facilitate discussion of current strategies used to increase their participation in medical education, and explore new strategies along the educational and professional pipeline that may have potential to increase participation in medicine,

---

[5] For the full report, see https://members.aamc.org/eweb/upload/Black_Males_in_Medicine_Report_WEB.pdf (accessed March 15, 2018).

[6] See also Institute of Medicine. 2003. *Unequal treatment: Confronting racial and ethnic disparities in health care.* Washington, DC: The National Academies Press. https://www.nap.edu/catalog/10260 (accessed March 20, 2018).

[7] Laurencin is university professor, Van Dusen Distinguished Professor of Orthopaedic Surgery, and director, The Raymond and Beverly Sackler Center at the University of Connecticut.

[8] Murray is state treatment coordinator/research assistant at UConn Health.

[9] For the paper, see https://link.springer.com/article/10.1007%2Fs40615-017-0380-y (accessed April 4, 2018) and https://nam.edu/an-american-crisis-the-lack-of-black-men-in-medicine (accessed April 4, 2018).

> **BOX 1-1**
> **Statement of Task**
>
> An ad hoc committee will plan and conduct a 2-day public workshop that will feature invited presentations and discussions that will explore the factors that contribute to low African American male participation in the medical profession, the current strategies used to increase participation in medical education, and new strategies that may have the potential to increase participation.
>
> The committee will define the specific topics to be addressed, develop the agenda, and select and invite speakers and other participants. A proceedings of the joint workshop will be prepared by a designated rapporteur in accordance with institutional guidelines.
>
> This workshop is joint with the W. Montague Cobb/NMA Health Institute (Cobb Institute), whose aim is to develop, evaluate, and implement strategies to promote wellness and eliminate health disparities and racism in medicine.

the Health and Medicine Division of the National Academies of Sciences, Engineering, and Medicine (the National Academies) and the Cobb Institute jointly convened a 2-day workshop on November 20 and 21, 2017, in Washington, DC.

An ad hoc committee (see Box 1-1 for the planning committee's Statement of Task) planned and designed the workshop to meet the following objectives:

- Briefly review the past and current history of Black men in medicine and science and the challenges encountered in the transition points to becoming successful physicians and scientists.
- Explore innovative strategies to support entry and successful passage through educational and career transition points leading to an increase in Black men in science and medicine.
- Consider the role of government, educational systems, philanthropy, industry, and others in effecting change along educational transition points.
- Explore ways in which innovative strategies can be shared with others, spread, and scaled up.

To achieve these objectives, the planning committee organized panels addressing challenges and barriers for Black men's entry into the medical profession, current strategies to address these challenges, and how medical schools, philanthropies, and government can address the absence of Black men in medicine.

OPENING REMARKS

In his introductory comments at the workshop, J. Michael McGinnis, M.D., M.P.P.,[10] noted that the absence of Black men in medicine is a problem not only for health and medicine, but a challenge for the future leadership of society at large. NAM President Dzau was unable to attend the meeting in person, but sent a recorded video providing some context about diversity in medical education. In his recorded remarks, he noted that African Americans, Latinos, and Native Americans are underrepresented in the health professions relative to their proportion of the U.S. population. Drawing on *Missing Persons: Minorities in the Health Professions*,[11] the 2004 Sullivan Commission on Diversity in the Healthcare Workforce report, which keynote speaker Sullivan chaired, Dzau added that enrollments of racial and ethnic minorities in medical, dental, and nursing schools are projected to decline. Dzau commented that he hoped that the workshop would serve as a "call to action to all of us to work together to reverse these trends." He stated that the shortage of Black men in medicine is of particular concern given the poorer health outcomes they experience relative to other racial, ethnic, and gender groups in the United States. He elaborated that this shortage "threatens the quality of our health system, hampers progress improving health for all, and challenges equity and justice."

Laurencin pointed out that the dearth of Black men in medicine is not a new issue, but a growing issue. He highlighted the article he coauthored with Murray on this issue, which they describe as "an American crisis that threatens efforts to effectively address health disparities, and to address excellence in clinical care."[12] He closed his remarks by echoing Dzau's hope that the meeting would be a "call to arms for people to get together nationally to move forward." He elaborated that the workshop is intended to bring out ideas. Additionally, he commented that the proceedings of the workshop could be used as a tool to discuss the ideas raised at the meeting and to raise awareness about the growing absence of Black men in medicine as a problem for all Americans.

ORGANIZATION OF THE PROCEEDINGS

This Proceedings of a Joint Workshop describes presentations, synthesizes discussions that occurred at the workshop, and highlights par-

---

[10] McGinnis is Leonard D. Schaeffer Executive Officer and Senior Scholar at the NAM.

[11] For more information, see http://www.aacnnursing.org/Portals/42/Diversity/SullivanReport.pdf (accessed February 20, 2018).

[12] For more information, see https://nam.edu/an-american-crisis-the-lack-of-Black-men-in-medicine (accessed February 20, 2018).

ticipants' ideas for opportunities that may have potential to address the absence of Black men in medicine. Chapter 2 summarizes two keynote presentations that examine the history and current state of Black men in medicine, the problem of their growing absence, and why it matters for health and health care. Chapter 3 summarizes presentations on the challenges and barriers Black men face along the life trajectory that may contribute to their absence in the health professions, while the presentations in Chapter 4 focus on challenges and barriers along the educational trajectory. Chapter 5 examines current strategies to support the entry of Black men in medicine. Chapter 6 summarizes reflections on the barriers for Black men to pursue medical careers and the current strategies to address them from the first day of the meeting. Chapter 7 begins with opening remarks from the second day of the meeting and discusses how medical schools can increase diversity in their student body and how they can hold themselves accountable for doing so. The presentations in Chapter 8 examine financial barriers to medical education, including how non-educational financial cost can hinder educational achievements. Chapter 9 summarizes presentations on the role of philanthropies, and Chapter 10 discusses the role of government. Chapter 11 presents final reflections on the workshop sessions and summarizes a general discussion in which participants brainstormed potential strategies to address the dearth of Black men in medicine.

In accordance with the policies of the National Academies workshop participants did not attempt to establish any conclusions or recommendations about needs and future directions, focusing instead on issues discussed by the speakers and workshop participants. In addition, the planning committee's role was limited to planning the workshop. Cato T. Laurencin was the designated rapporteur and prepared a factual summary of what occurred at the workshop.

2

Keynote Presentations

As a basis for the workshop's discussions, two keynote speakers provided an overview of the history and current status of Black men in medicine and the consequences of this problem on the health care workforce and on health outcomes. Louis Sullivan, M.D., provided a historical perspective, reviewing key policies and practices that contributed to the present shortage of Black men in medicine, and described the adverse consequences on health outcomes and health disparities. Darrell G. Kirch, M.D., provided a broader health care context for the issue, describing what he identified as four serious challenges in health care that, to address, require inclusion and, moreover, solving the problem of the shortage of Black men in medicine. Following the presentations, George C. Hill, Ph.D.,[1] moderated a brief discussion.

[1] Sullivan is chairman and chief executive officer of The Sullivan Alliance to Transform the Health Professions and president emeritus of the Morehouse School of Medicine. Kirch is president and chief executive officer of the American Association of Medical Colleges (AAMC). Hill is Levi Watkins Jr., M.D. professor emeritus in medical education, distinguished professor emeritus in the Department of Pathology, Microbiology, and Immunology, and past vice chancellor for equity, diversity and inclusion and chief diversity officer at Vanderbilt University.

OPENING KEYNOTE

Louis Sullivan, M.D.
Chairman and Chief Executive Officer
The Sullivan Alliance to Transform the Health Professions
President Emeritus
Morehouse School of Medicine

Sullivan began by describing how a history of slavery, segregation, discrimination, and bias (both conscious and unconscious) resulted in "less opportunity for Blacks and greater poverty in America's Black population." He then described the influence of Abraham Flexner's 1910 report *Medical Education in the United States and Canada*,[2] which recommended the closure of certain medical schools owing to the inadequate faculty, weak curriculum, and low standards. The report resulted in the closure of many medical schools by 1925, including five of the seven predominantly Black medical schools, leaving Howard University College of Medicine and Meharry Medical College as the only predominantly Black medical schools in the first half of the 20th century.

Sullivan continued by discussing the convergence of an expansion of medical education and the Civil Rights movement in the latter half of the 20th century, which resulted in increasing opportunity for Black men in medicine. Sullivan identified several key contributions to this convergence. First, the Supreme Court decision in *Brown v. Board of Education* in 1954 resulted in the integration of medical schools. Second, two predominantly Black medical schools, the Morehouse School of Medicine and the Charles R. Drew University of Medicine and Science, were established. Third, in 1986, the AAMC launched study committees to increase racial and ethnic diversity in medical schools, which issued several recommendations, including broadening and strengthening the educational pipeline.

Next, Sullivan elaborated on the contraction of opportunity for Black men to enter health professions in the United States since the 1980s. He pointed out that a perceived surplus of doctors resulted in the end of the era of expansion for medical schools, and highlighted how decreased state and federal funding for medical education has led to significant increases in tuition for health professional schools, which in turn has contributed to the growing burden of educational debt. He noted that this potential burden may be a financial barrier for racial and ethnic minority students to enter medical school. He added that although the average debt at

[2] For more information, see http://archive.carnegiefoundation.org/pdfs/elibrary/Carnegie_Flexner_Report.pdf (accessed February 20, 2018).

graduation has more than doubled in three decades, the proportion of medical students graduating without debt has increased from 16 percent to 27 percent.[3] He commented that this suggests that the proportion of affluent medical students is increasing. Finally, Sullivan described the 2015 AAMC report *Altering the Course: Black Males in Medicine*,[4] which highlighted the failure to increase the number of Black men applying to and entering medical school. Sullivan remarked that, although the number of Black medical students increased overall between 1978 and 2014, gains in representation among Black women were primarily responsible for this overall increase. During the same period, the number of Black male students entering medical schools *decreased* by 25 percent.

Having provided historical context for the absence of Black men in medicine, Sullivan proceeded to discuss why this absence is problematic—or, why it matters. First, he said, it reflects a lack of opportunity for racial and ethnic minorities to become health professionals, "depriving the nation of the contributions [these individuals] could make to improve their lives, their community, and their country." Citing a *New England Journal of Medicine* study by Komaromy and colleagues, Sullivan added that a less diverse health care workforce contributes to the poorer access to health services that racial and ethnic minorities, individuals with low socioeconomic position, and those living in geographically remote areas experience.[5] Furthermore, Sullivan noted that less diversity is also likely to result in a less culturally competent health care workforce. He continued to explain that decreased access to health care services and receipt of lower quality health care in turn contribute to the poorer health status of African Americans. Moreover, he argued that a non-diverse health workforce is a problem for the country as a whole. Sullivan quoted from a 2016 *Health Affairs* article he authored:

> When minority students give up their dream of becoming a doctor or other health professional, they are depriving themselves; depriving future patients who would benefit from having a more ethnically and racially diverse health care workforce; and depriving the nation of the

[3] See Grischkan, J., B. P. George, K. Chaiyachati, A. B. Friedman, E. R. Dorsey, and D. A. Asch. 2017. Distribution of medical education debt by specialty, 2010–2016. *JAMA Internal Medicine* 177(10):1532–1535. https://jamanetwork.com/journals/jamainternalmedicine/fullarticle/2652831 (accessed April 27, 2018).

[4] For more information, see https://members.aamc.org/eweb/upload/Altering%20the%20Course%20-%20Black%20Males%20in%20Medicine%20AAMC.pdf (accessed February 20, 2018).

[5] For more information, see Komaromy, M., K. Grumbach, M. Drake, K. Vranizan, N. Lurie, D. Keane, and A. B. Bindman. 1996. The role of Black and Hispanic physicians in providing health care for underserved populations. *New England Journal of Medicine* 334:1305–1310. https://www.nejm.org/doi/full/10.1056/NEJM199605163342006 (accessed May 3, 2018).

contributions they could make to improving their lives, their community, and the country. (p. 1534)[6]

Sullivan closed his talk by challenging his audience:

> All of us are challenged to find better answers, better approaches to these challenges, and to find more effective solutions to increase diversity in the health professions. . . . It is up to you, and to me, to provide encouragement and leadership and have others join us in this effort. That is a challenge. We must plan, we must educate and engage our colleagues, then forge ahead. The health of our increasingly diverse nation depends upon it. Our commitment of our society to fairness and equal opportunity demands it. It is up to you and me to see that that happens.

THE PERSPECTIVE FROM ACADEMIC MEDICINE

Darrell G. Kirch, M.D.
President and Chief Executive Officer
Association of American Medical Colleges

Kirch began by reviewing the AAMC's role in promoting a diverse medical workforce. He recalled the history of the AAMC and its evolution in supporting diversity and inclusion in medicine. Like much of the nation, the AAMC's past on the issue demonstrates significant change toward progress. For example, in 1950, W. Montague Cobb asked the association's leadership to make a statement against discrimination and segregation in medical schools. The AAMC Executive Council noted that while it gave sympathetic consideration to the question presented by Dr. Cobb, the AAMC reaffirmed its traditional position that it is not within the scope of this association to take action on matters that are within the jurisdiction of the individual medical school and a matter of internal administration within that school. Kirch went on to describe the evolution of the AAMC since that time to promote diversity and inclusion, which includes establishing an Office of Minority Affairs and, in 1991, launching the 3000 by 2000 project, a national campaign that aimed to enroll 3,000 underrepresented racial and ethnic minority students in medical school by the year 2000.[7] Finally, he presented selected statistics about Black men in medicine, updated from the 2015 AAMC report *Altering the Course:*

---

[6] To read the *Health Affairs* article, see https://www.healthaffairs.org/doi/abs/10.1377/hlthaff.2016.0382 (accessed February 27, 2018).

[7] For more information, see http://www.jdentaled.org/content/67/9/1048.long (accessed February 27, 2018).

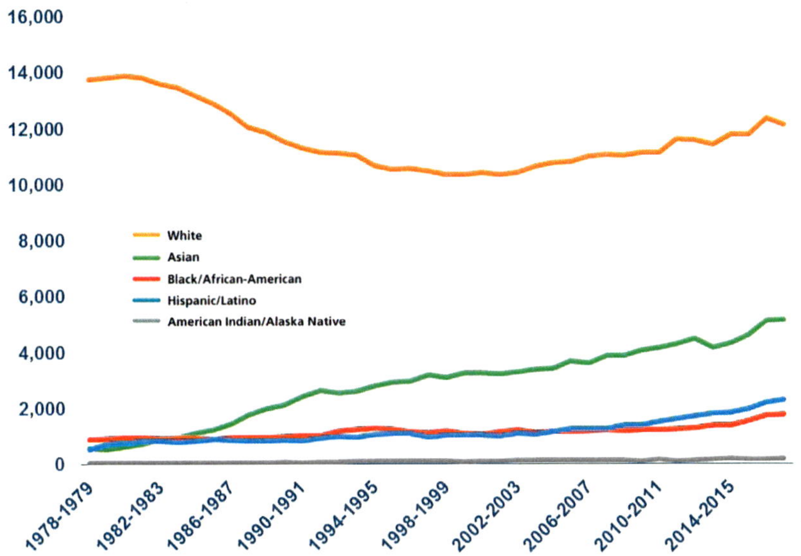

FIGURE 2-1 Matriculants to U.S. medical schools by race/ethnicity (alone or in combination), 1978–1979 through 2017–2018, as of November 1, 2017.
SOURCES: Kirch presentation, November 20, 2017. Data from AAMC, 2017.

Black Males in Medicine, which Sullivan also cited.[8] Adding to Sullivan's comments on the report in his keynote address, Kirch noted that there has been only a modest increase in the number of Black or African American matriculants to U.S. medical schools since 1978 (see Figure 2-1). With respect to Black men in particular, in 2017, less than 40 percent of those applicants matriculated to medical school. Additionally, although there is near parity of men and women for many racial and ethnic groups, Black or African American matriculants are 61 percent women compared with just 39 percent men (see Figure 2-2).

Kirch then focused his presentation on what he described as four serious challenges for health care. He noted that inclusion is key among the solutions to these challenges, including solving the problem of low participation of Black men in medicine. First, he said, health care reimbursement and delivery are changing rapidly, which requires care models that employ clinician teams. He added that diversity and inclusion

[8] For more information, see https://members.aamc.org/eweb/upload/Altering%20the%20Course%20-%20Black%20Males%20in%20Medicine%20AAMC.pdf (accessed February 20, 2018).

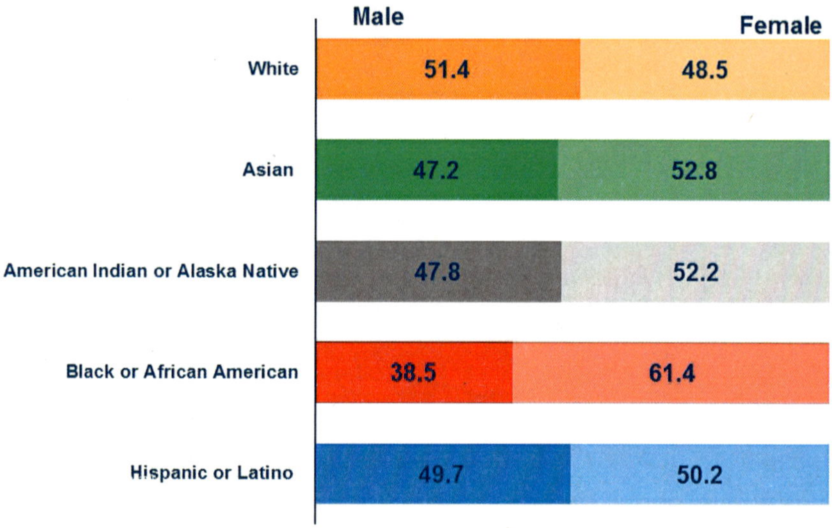

FIGURE 2-2 Matriculants to U.S. medical schools by race/ethnicity (alone or in combination) and sex, 2016–2017 and 2017–2018, as of November 1, 2017.
SOURCES: Kirch presentation, November 20, 2017. Data from AAMC, 2017.

are critical to effective teamwork, because, "A team will always solve a problem much better than an individual, and a diverse team will solve a problem much better, much faster than a homogeneous team." Kirch identified clinician burnout and resilience as the second major challenge, and remarked, "Inclusive work environments . . . help foster resilience and well-being and combat burnout."

He then described the phenomenon of the "minority tax." As described in a 2017 article by Kali D. Cyrus in the *Journal of the American Medical Association*, the minority tax is "the additional responsibilities placed on minority faculty to achieve diversity" or "the expectation [that minority faculty] represent [their] otherness across the institution for the good of the community, often at the expense of the individual."[9] Kirch suggested that the minority tax, in addition to all other causal factors, may contribute to burnout among racial and ethnic minority learners, faculty, and staff. The third challenge Kirch identified was leadership—in particular, the need for a more diverse pool of leaders and for a different

[9] For more information on the minority tax, see https://bmcmededuc.biomedcentral.com/articles/10.1186/s12909-015-0290-9 (accessed February 21, 2018) and https://jamanetwork.com/journals/jama/fullarticle/2625322 (accessed February 21, 2018).

kind of leader. He described a shift from an outdated model of leaders as "Moses," in which the leader is a "genius coming down from the mountaintop," to a leader as a "multiplier . . . who can most effectively activate the genius of all those around him or her."[10] He elaborated that the new leadership model requires the ability to change culture.

The final challenge Kirch identified was the need to achieve a truly holistic selection process for admission into medical school. This requires a shift from traditional criteria such as test scores and grades to different competencies, including academic readiness (i.e., traditional competences in scientific knowledge and quantitative reasoning), diversity, and "preprofessional readiness." The latter encompasses skills and attributes the AAMC collectively refers to as "15 Core Competencies for Entering Medical Students," including cultural competence, critical thinking, resilience and adaptability, social skills, teamwork and communications skills, ethical responsibility, and a capacity for improvement.

Kirch closed his presentation with a reminder that the goal of promoting a diverse health care workforce is to improve health equity. Furthermore, he asserted that beyond health, "We need to counter the deep and in some ways growing divisions and injustices that exist in our country and our health system." He elaborated that academic health centers can serve as a place to bring communities together and "accomplish social repair."

DISCUSSION

Cedric M. Bright, M.D., FACP,[11] asked about the role of scholarship in financing medical education, especially in light of the fact that, as Sullivan mentioned, affluent students comprise an increasingly greater share of medical students. Sullivan remarked that the idea that medical students will become high-earning physicians who can quickly repay their loans with future earnings no longer holds true for many students, and declared the need to counter this assumption. In so doing, he suggested a reframing of the issue of medical education financing as a social problem rather than an individual problem. He said, "We as a society need physicians and other health professionals in the same way we need engineers and lawyers. I see this as an investment in our society." Kirch suggested a need to reframe how schools think about scholarship, citing "Is There Merit

---

[10] For more information on multipliers, see Wiseman, L. 2010. *Multipliers: How the best leaders make everyone smarter*. New York: HarperCollins.

[11] Bright is associate dean for inclusive excellence, director of the Office of Special Programs, and associate professor of medicine at the University of North Carolina School of Medicine.

in Merit Aid?" a *New England Journal of Medicine* article.[12] In summarizing the author's points, he commented, "Schools pursuing scholarships oriented towards academic merit often favor the fairly affluent, which may be subverting our desire to bring in a broader socioeconomic and diverse class." In closing, Sullivan put forward the need to increase public awareness, advocate for policy issues beyond health and medicine, restore trust in civic institutions, cultivate leadership that collaborates and works together, and rally public support around medical education financing. He said,

> What we need to do is develop a community of leaders, both in the public sector and the private sector, to educate the public about this. What we need is public support. . . . It's not something that an individual can do. We need to have teams of people doing it, but if we are the core, if that is to happen, we're the ones that have to make it happen.

[12] See http://www.nejm.org/doi/full/10.1056/NEJMp1713146 (accessed February 27, 2018).

3

Exploring the Challenges and Barriers for Black Men Along the Life Trajectory

Highlights Presented by Individual Speakers

- Racism is a fundamental cause of the low priority of addressing the underrepresentation of Black men in medicine. (Jones)
- By examining how racism is operating with regard to the shortage of Black men in medicine, it is possible to identify mechanisms that can be targeted for intervention to increase representation of Black men in medicine. (Jones)
- Addressing the lack of Black men in medicine requires acknowledging and improving the social and environmental factors around some Black men and boys. (Mitchell)
- Early access and exposure to science, technology, engineering, and mathematics (STEM) education, mentoring, and having a "mirror of relevance" can promote positive self-image among young Black men and help them see themselves as physicians. (Mitchell)
- Mental health and behavioral challenges (including substance use) hinder Black male educational attainment. (Evans)
- A population health approach to behavioral health care may better meet the needs of Black boys and men and thus improve their health and life outcomes. (Evans)

- Psychological factors such as the beliefs and expectations of others, self-perceptions, self-efficacy, and perceived racism can be barriers to entering the medical profession among Black boys and men. (Evans)
- Mentoring, strengthening social support networks, and addressing perceived discrimination can help Black boys and men overcome psychological barriers to becoming physicians. (Evans)
- The lack of Black men in medicine is a problem in need of an urgent solution. (Jones)

The first panel of the workshop featured presentations on the barriers and challenges Black boys and men face across their life spans. The panel especially focused on circumstances and events outside of the educational system that can influence their achievement. Camara Jones, M.D., M.P.H., Ph.D., described racism as a fundamental root cause of the lack of Black men in medicine. Drawing from his own experience, Roger Mitchell, Jr., M.D., described the importance of role models and socioenvironmental barriers, such as mass incarceration and unsafe and underresourced neighborhood environments. Arthur C. Evans, Jr., Ph.D., discussed psychological issues that are barriers for Black men to entering medical careers. Wizdom Powell, Ph.D., led a brief discussion following the presentations.[1]

RACISM

Camara Jones, M.D., M.P.H., Ph.D.
Senior Fellow
Satcher Health Leadership Institute
Morehouse School of Medicine

Racism is a system of power that structures opportunity and assigns value, and which can occur via acts of commission or acts of omission (such as inaction in the face of need), Jones began. She described the low prioritization of the shortage of Black men in medicine as an act of omission and a form of racism and defined racism on three levels—institutionalized, personally mediated, and internalized racism. Institutionalized racism is the

[1] Jones is senior fellow at the Satcher Health Leadership Institute at Morehouse School of Medicine. Mitchell is chief medical examiner for the District of Columbia. Evans is chief executive officer of the American Psychological Association. Powell is director of the Health Disparities Institute at UConn Health.

"constellation of structures, policies, practices, norms, and values that taken together result in differential access to the goods, services, and opportunities of society by race." Examples of these goods, services, and opportunities include

- Housing
- Education
- Employment
- Income
- Medical facilities
- Clean environment
- Information

Jones also described valuing people differently by race and ethnicity and the disproportionate incarceration of racial and ethnic minorities as examples. Personally mediated racism refers to "differential assumptions about the abilities, motives, and intents of others by race, and then differential actions based on those assumptions." It also captures discrimination, prejudice, and conscious and unconscious bias. Jones identified several examples of personally mediated racism, including

- Police brutality
- Physician disrespect
- Shopkeeper vigilance
- Waiter indifference
- Teacher devaluation

Internalized racism is the "acceptance by members of stigmatized races of negative messages about our own abilities and intrinsic worth . . . accepting limitations to [our] full humanity of the box into which [we have] been placed." Examples of internalized racism include

- Self-devaluation
- Resignation
- Helplessness
- Hopelessness

Jones continued by briefly presenting the Gardener's Tale, an allegory about a gardener with two flower boxes, one with rich soil and one with poor soil, and red and pink flowers. The allegory illustrates the three levels of racism and is a tool to provide a common language to understand racism, to talk about racism, and to structure how to think about intervening to mitigate the influence of racism on health. In this allegory, the gardener represents the government or those with power to make decisions and to act, as well as who controls access to resources. The flower boxes represent structural factors that separate rich soil (advantaged environments) from poor soil (disadvantaged environments). The flower colors represent traits (e.g., race). The gardener's preference for red flowers over pink represents normative aspects of institutionalized racism.[2] Using this allegory, Jones underscored the importance of understanding how racism is operating with respect to the dearth of Black men in medicine. She explained,

> But we need to know how [to] answer the question, "How is racism operating here?" It is a system with identifiable mechanisms that are in our structures, policies, practices, norms, and values. Different aspects of decision making structures are the who, what, when, and where of decision making. Who is at the table and who is not? How are the policies written? What are the unwritten practices and norms? How and why do we assign values?

Jones finished her presentation by identifying potential mechanisms of racism that could be targets for interventions to increase the number of Black men in medicine. Some of these mechanisms are

- The medical education pipeline as a structure,
- Funding public education through property taxes as a policy,
- The lack of Black faculty and community members on medical school admissions committees as a practice,
- The shortage of Black men in medicine not being understood as a societal problem requiring an urgent solution as a norm, and
- The view of Black men as inherently threatening as a value.

REFLECTIONS ON BARRIERS TO BECOMING A PHYSICIAN

Roger Mitchell, Jr., M.D.
Chief Medical Examiner
District of Columbia

Mitchell reflected on his own experience becoming a physician and as a medical examiner to identify potential barriers to medical education. Mitchell began by describing the "heavy backpack" of social factors young Black men carry. These challenges include

---

[2] To read Jones's Gardener's Tale, see http://ajph.aphapublications.org/doi/pdf/10.2105/AJPH.90.8.1212 (accessed February 21, 2018).

- Difficult social and familial relationships,
- Interactions with the criminal justice system, and
- Living in neighborhoods high in violence and low in socioeconomic position and educational opportunity.

Mitchell identified several actions that could address these negative influences on Black boys and young men to help them pursue medical education and careers. First, Mitchell encouraged the audience to promote access and exposure to science, technology, engineering, and medical (STEM) education from a young age. Second, Mitchell highlighted the importance of role models and having a "mirror of relevance." He asserted,

> That mirror of relevance is extremely important, to put that up in front of other Black men that you want to become physicians. They have to see it as relevant to who they are and who their culture is.

Mitchell elaborated that providing role models could facilitate changing "the narrative of who Black men are" by changing norms and values, especially on Black boys and young men's own expectations and aspirations. Finally, he encouraged action to address the social and environmental factors around some Black boys and men to help these boys and men to develop a positive self-narrative, "to create an environment where they can see themselves as physicians."

MENTAL HEALTH AND RESILIENCY IN THE LIVES OF BLACK MEN

Arthur C. Evans, Jr., Ph.D.
Chief Executive Officer
American Psychological Association

Evans began by describing mental health disparities experienced by Black men. He proposed that understanding health care disparities is important for understanding not only the health of Black men, but also other life outcomes, including higher rates of incarceration and worse educational outcomes. He commented, "If you care about the pipeline of African American men and boys being available to go into careers in science and in medicine, you have to care about behavioral health challenges." He added that, importantly, although the prevalence of serious mental illnesses is similar among Black men compared with women and other racial and ethnic groups, how these illnesses play out differs greatly. He offered that the different outcomes can be attributed to increased exposure to violence and to barriers to care. He expanded that addressing these barriers to care and thereby improving life outcomes among Black men therefore requires a systems change, and proposed re-conceptualizing behavioral health care.

The next part of Evans's presentation focused on how the behavioral health care system can better meet the needs of Black boys and men to improve their health and life outcomes. He continued with what he described as two major problems with the current health care system. First, he said individuals with severe or even diagnosable mental and behavioral health challenges comprise only a small portion of the total population. He added that even in the majority of the population considered to be healthy, some may have subclinical issues that will quickly develop into a mental disorder above the diagnostic threshold, but for which no mechanisms or resources to deal with them exist. Second, he said that although resources are heavily focused on the provision of health care, many other factors (such as social determinants of health) influence health status and remain unaddressed. Thus, he proposed the need for a population health approach to behavioral health care. Such an approach targets healthy individuals and those at risk for disease (i.e., those with undiagnosed or subclinical mental health issues) and not merely those with severe mental illness or a diagnosable mental disorder.

For those at risk of developing mental health disorders, such as those who have experienced trauma either directly or vicariously, Evans proposed the need for evidence-based treatments. As an example, Evans offered screening children for traumatic stress in pediatric settings. Second, Evans proposed the need to change norms about mental health, especially among Black men and described the "Engaging Males of Color" initiative to "get men to reframe and think about their mental wellness differently," such as by changing the language through storytelling.

Beyond the clinical disorders and care, Evans discussed the need to "address the psychological barriers [to entering the mental health professions], anticipate them, start much earlier . . . in elementary school, and follow kids all the way through the educational pipeline into [health professional] careers." These psychological factors include the beliefs and expectations of others, self-perceptions, self-efficacy, and perceived racism. He proposed ways to address these psychological barriers such as through "mentorship programs . . . [to] help people navigate through the educational system, building broader networks of social support." He also proposed addressing perceived discrimination such as by promoting a strong and positive racial identity and promoting resilience. Finally, Evans discussed the need for research on these mental and behavioral issues.

DISCUSSION

Valerie Montgomery Rice, M.D.,[3] posed a question about resilience, asking whether any current research seeks to identify characteristics that have helped Black male physicians to succeed despite the barriers and challenges they faced. She suggested that looking at positive characteristics associated with success rather than just focusing on negative challenges and barriers to achievement may be important. Evans responded that resilience is an emerging but growing area of research and echoed the need for more research. Jones cautioned against focusing on resilience as an individual characteristic at the expense of seeking structural solutions. Using the allegory of the Gardener's Tale, she said:

> Although resilience is very important, we need to be attentive to the soil [or, structures and environment]. Because if you talk about the resilient ones, sometimes it's a counterexample: "Well, this one made it despite that, so you should just try harder." . . . [This is] a variation in the strength of the seed [i.e., individual differences]. But what we need to do is have such rich soil that you don't have to be that superstar or whatever to make it, just like you don't have the red seed [a member of a privileged group]. . . . I think that resilience is important in the short term, but if it diverts our attention from addressing the quality of the soil, then it could actually do us a disservice.

Responding to Jones's comment, a participant offered that the choice between examining resilience as an individual characteristic and structural barriers need not be binary. The participant asserted,

> What we assume is that there are superstars. And what I'm saying is that a lot of people are not superstars, and they all have the same soil. So there's something else that's going on. We from a research perspective need to begin to look at what that something else is.

Mitchell echoed the sentiments of this participant, offering that, based on his own experience of becoming a doctor, resilience may be a product of the individual and the environment in which he is embedded and "many of us know intuitively or through our own experience what [that resiliency] was." However, research to quantify and qualify that subjective experience of resilience through rigorous research would be welcome.

---

[3] Montgomery Rice is president and dean of the Morehouse School of Medicine.

Reflecting on Jones's definition of racism, Cato T. Laurencin, M.D., Ph.D.,[4] emphasized that racism "is an assignment of value [and] the creation of these different structures . . . is justified on the basis of inferiority of Black people." Jones expanded on this comment, suggesting a need to look at how "white supremacist ideology [and] cultural racism" as societal values that structure society are fundamental drivers of the problem of a shortage of Black men in medicine. She elaborated on the importance of calling out this racism as "a problem requiring urgent solution" and added that, without addressing this fundamental cause, the system of medical education will continue to disadvantage Black students while privileging students of other races and ethnicities regardless of the pipeline programs implemented to mitigate the effects of this racism on the representation of Black men in medicine.

[4] Laurencin is university professor, Van Dusen Distinguished Professor of Orthopaedic Surgery, and director, The Raymond and Beverly Sackler Center at the University of Connecticut.

4

Exploring the Challenges and Barriers for Black Men Along the Educational Trajectory

Highlights Presented by Individual Speakers

- Lack of educational and financial resources and lack of confidence (or, negative self-perception and low self-efficacy) are primary barriers to achieving medical careers among Black boys and men. (Holden)
- Community colleges are an underused resource; these schools have students that can be used to build the pool of Black men and students of color in medicine and can serve as a hub for community collaboration to strengthen the medical education pipeline and to support students in the pipeline. (Moore)
- Medical educational pipeline programs need to appeal to students' interest in science, technology, engineering, and mathematics (STEM) careers. (Verret)
- Medical educational pipeline programs need to start early in the pipeline—in elementary and middle school. (Verret)
- Disparities in public education leave Black boys less prepared for pursuing medicine in higher education. (Verret)
- Classroom behaviors that used to be considered normal are now diagnosed as illness and medicated; alternately, these behaviors are considered criminal and divert students to the criminal justice system through the school-to-prison pipeline. (Verret)

- Black men are underrepresented in all areas of academia, not just in medicine. (Britt)
- Addressing the shortage of Black men in medicine will require partnerships with a broad range of stakeholders, generating specific action items and not just talk, and cultivating a culture of financial stability and sustainability for financing medical education. (Britt)

The second panel of the meeting examined challenges and barriers for Black boys and men across academia, from elementary education to medical school and on through medical residency and academic careers. Lynne Holden, M.D.,[1] presented the nationwide Mentoring in Medicine program she developed, which provides mentoring and support to students from elementary through health professional schools. Walter J. Lanier, J.D.,[2] presented the Men of Color initiative he created at the Milwaukee Area Technical College (MATC), which aims to increase course completion, retention, and graduation rates among men of color at the college. C. Reynold Verret, Ph.D., president of Xavier University of Louisiana, describes how Xavier successfully produces the greatest number of Black physicians compared with other schools across the country. L. D. Britt, M.D.,[3] presented observations from his career as a mentor and educator to Black men pursuing medical professions. The session was moderated by Marc Nivet, Ed.D.,[4] who proposed in his opening remarks that the only way to effectively increase the number of African American medical students is to open up more African American medical schools and to increase the number of African American seats in all medical schools. Nivet led a brief discussion following the presentations.

[1] Holden is president and chief executive officer of Mentoring in Medicine, emergency department physician and residency site director of the Emergency Medicine Residency Program at Montefiore Medical Center, and associate professor of clinical emergency medicine at the Albert Einstein College of Medicine.

[2] Lanier is director of multicultural affairs and community engagement at the Milwaukee Area Technical College.

[3] Britt is Henry Ford Professor and Edward J. Brickhouse Chairman at Eastern Virginia Medical School.

[4] Nivet is executive vice president for institutional advancement at UT Southwestern Medical Center.

MENTORING IN MEDICINE

Lynne Holden, M.D.
President and Chief Executive Officer
Mentoring in Medicine

Holden first presented the Mentoring in Medicine program, reviewing its history, mission, and programs. Mentoring in Medicine offers school-based programs, which provide a daily elective class in low-resource inner city schools for students beginning in the second grade, and out-of-school camps that occur throughout the calendar year, which include virtual programming to reach students across the country. For college and postbaccalaureate students, Mentoring in Medicine offers programs with clinical exposure, internships, and seminars. The organization also has a "Parents STEM Network," which provides in-house and virtual networking opportunities to help parents better understand the challenges their children face while studying STEM. Since its founding in 2008, Mentoring in Medicine has seen 176 of its students accepted and matriculating to 37 medical schools. Holden commented that all of these students were discouraged from applying to medical school.[5]

Based on interviews with students, parents, and educators, Holden and colleagues identified three primary barriers. They found the principal barrier was that a lack of confidence, or the self-perception that "they don't have the resources. No one looks like me who is doing this." The second biggest barrier they identified was a lack of educational resources. Financial resources came third (Holden et al., 2014).

Finally, Holden presented lessons learned, beginning with the need for a team to help students overcome psychological barriers. Holden stated,

> You really have to erase a lot of pressures, a lot of everyday what's happening in their environment, and you have to paint a different picture, a different movie. It takes a team of people to do that. It takes social workers, psychologists—it takes mentors. It just takes a lot of people to make it happen.

She added, "You have to make sure that you appeal to the heart. Let them be leaders. Whatever they learn, let them do it. Let them tell and share with their communities."

[5] For more information about Mentoring in Medicine, see http://medicalmentor.org (accessed February 26, 2018).

MEN OF COLOR

Walter J. Lanier, J.D.
Director of Multicultural Affairs and Community Engagement
Milwaukee Area Technical College

Lanier opened his presentation by highlighting the importance of community colleges as an underused resource. In his words,

> The community college is kind of a hidden jewel, a hidden resource, a hidden, naturally occurring pool in the educational ecosystem. We just miss it. There is already a bridge; there is already a body of people in the ecosystem of the community college that we can use to build this pool of Black men and students of color in medicine.

For context, Lanier commented that in 2014, of all Black undergraduate students, 44 percent were in community colleges.[6] At the MATC, he said, 56 percent of students identify as a racial or ethnic minority, and 22 percent of students identify as men of color.

Lanier then described the Men of Color Initiative at the MATC,[7] which offers a range of strategies to increase course completion, retention, and graduation/program completion, and to close equity gaps. These strategies include building cohorts, partnering with academic programs, community collaborations, aggressive data use to identify targets for intervention, promoting health and wellness, providing mentoring and role modeling, and offering professional development. The initiative also surveys students for input about their needs from their perspective.

To illustrate the potential of community colleges and describe the application of some of the Men of Color Initiative strategies, Lanier discussed a mental health awareness day hosted by MATC that brought together stakeholders including religious organizations, local health systems and health services agencies, local law firms, and advocacy organizations. He remarked,

> It was a deep community collaborative to take the messages [of academia] and embed it inside the community college to propagate it broadly to our community . . . what made it catalytic was doing it at the community college, which is an institution that, as part of its mission, is connected to the ground.

---

[6] See https://trends.collegeboard.org/sites/default/files/trends-in-community-colleges-research-brief.pdf (accessed February 26, 2018).

[7] For more information about Men in Color at the MATC, see https://matcmenofcolor.wordpress.com/about (accessed February 27, 2018).

Lanier closed his presentation by challenging those in the room to think about the role community colleges can play in programs to strengthen the medical education pipeline.

CHALLENGES ALONG THE EDUCATIONAL PIPELINE

C. Reynold Verret, Ph.D.
President
Xavier University of Louisiana

Verret opened his presentation by emphasizing the need to understand the origins of the shortage of Black men in medicine. He proceeded to discuss barriers and faciliators along the educational pipeline from his experience. First, he emphasized the need for programs to appeal to students' interest in STEM careers to start earlier in the educational pipeline, and suggested targeting middle school. He commented that the focus on identifying talented STEM students in undergraduate programs is an outlier compared with other disciplines, saying

> Talent begins at [8, 9, 10, or 11 years old]. If you don't catch talent when it's at that point . . . it goes away and finds another place. If we are asking ourselves to make cellists or great pianists, I would not say let's find those 18-year-olds and make great musicians. That's the way it is with scientists and with those who go into the health professions.

Verret then discussed disparities in public education as a barrier, arguing,

> The majority of American children do not get the education they deserve. We tend to blame them for not achieving and not being prepared. They do not choose their schools any more than they choose their parents. But they are not prepared.

Contributing to this bifurcated educational system, Verret next identified the disproportionate pathologizing and criminalizing of behavior by race and gender in schools as a systemic challenge. These reflect systematic biases in the use of exclusionary discipline and referrals to special education services for Black students compared with students of other racial and ethnic groups and for boys compared with girls (Skiba et al., 2000, 2011; Wallace et al., 2008). Moreover, he noted, these students internalize the notion that they are damaged, with adverse consequences for their own norms and expectations. To that end, Verret argued for the need to change these norms and expectations, offering, "What students need is belief, the expectation to succeed."

IDEAS TO POTENTIALLY ADDRESS THE SHORTAGE OF BLACK MEN IN MEDICINE

L. D. Britt, M.D.
Henry Ford Professor and Edward J. Brickhouse Chairman
Eastern Virginia Medical School

Britt began his presentation by pointing out that not only is the underrepresentation of Black men a problem in medicine, but also that "at no level of advanced education is there a robust number of Black men on an enhanced education trajectory. . . . Black men are underrepresented on every level of academia." He declared that addressing this challenge requires effort, initiatives, and leadership. With respect to specific actions, Britt first emphasized the importance of partnerships with stakeholders, including those not in the health care sector. Some potential stakeholders he identified include the National Academy of Medicine, the American Association of Medical Colleges, the U.S. Department of Health and Human Services, the U.S. Department of Education, the associations at public and private secondary schools, churches and religious organizations, and community organizations. Second, Britt highlighted the need to "generate specific action items, not just talk about things that we all know." Examples of specific actions he listed include summer camps, medicine-themed fairs (akin to science fairs), and "creative systems of magnet schools." Third, he emphasized the need to cultivate a culture of financial stability and sustainability for financing medical education and proposed using foundation grants and loan forgiveness programs as possible strategies. Finally, echoing Nivet's opening remarks, Britt underscored the need to expand medical schools and increase the number of seats in schools and residencies available for Black men.

DISCUSSION

Tammy Mayo-Blake, M.Ed., of the Health Resources and Services Administration, commented on her previous experience as a K–12 teacher and school counselor during a time when there was a movement to increase girls' involvement in education. She noted that she was accountable for increasing their participation in her performance evaluation. Reflecting on the successes of that movement, she asked the deans of medical schools in the room whether there are specific conversations at their institutions to increase participation of African American boys going into science and medicine careers. Verret responded that, whereas the lack of participation of girls in K–12 education was understood as a problem, the low participation of Black boys may not be similarly understood as a problem because it is a consequence of a pedagogic approach that focuses on achieving "class control . . . how to manage the class, how to control groups." He asserted that this focus on control may lead to pathologizing and criminalizing Black boys' behavior and suggested that other approaches to teaching may better meet the needs of Black boys who may have different learning styles. Britt emphasized the need to dismiss certain myths about what education and skills are needed to become a doctor, which result in poor or inadequate counseling and may discourage certain students from pursuing the health professions. For example, he cited the myth that undergraduate students must major in a science to go to medical school.

Bonnie Mason, M.D.,[8] inquired about the high attrition rates of Black residents compared with residents from other racial and ethnic groups. She asked,

> When are the people in this room going to develop either a race curriculum, a health disparities curriculum, or a way for our students who are called "N"? The N-word is being used in the operating room. The students are being cast aside and left out of classrooms when a patient says, "I don't want to see you as a Black physician."

In response, Britt emphasized the need to promote inclusive environments in addition to increasing the diversity of medical students. He expanded on this, saying that simply having a more diverse student body is insufficient. Students from diverse backgrounds must also all feel welcome and included in their learning environments. Leon McDougle, M.D., M.P.H.,[9] expanded on Britt's comment, and suggested that accountability to promote diversity and inclusion in residencies can be built into accreditation standards. He stated that his institution is advocating for the Accreditation Council for Graduate Medical Education to adopt a standard for diversity and inclusion similar to the existing one for medical schools. His proposed standard stated,

> A residency training program has effective policies and practices in place and engages in ongoing systematic and focused recruitment and retention activities to receive mission-appropriate diversity outcomes for students, faculty, senior administration staff, and other relevant members of the academic community.

[8] Mason is orthopedic surgeon and founder of Nth Dimensions, a nonprofit dedicated to increasing health equity by increasing diversity in some medical specialties. For more information, see http://www.nthdimensions.org (accessed Febrruary 27, 2018).

[9] McDougle is chief diversity officer at The Ohio State University Wexner Medical Center.

Finally, William Owen, M.D., FACP,[10] emphasized the need for institutional leadership and commitment to diversity and inclusion.

Marja Hurley, M.D.,[11] questioned whether there are strategies to capture Black men who apply to medical schools who are not accepted, to encourage them to reapply, and to ensure that they are better prepared in their reapplication. Nivet commented that current strategies such as enrichment programs or a supplemental year are not enough. Verret described a program at Xavier University of Louisiana in which students can take courses and be involved in research for a fifth year. Cato T. Laurencin, M.D., Ph.D.,[12] emphasized that this is a large group of untapped potential, and reiterated the need to first identify these students, "to get their names." Second, he suggested the need to develop a "pathway or program that allows their reentry."

Cedric M. Bright, M.D., FACP,[13] asked the panelists when and how they discuss racism with their students. He also inquired about strategies to discuss racism in a way that students "maintain that positive self-image before it becomes totally torn down because they start to buy into that stereotype threat."

Holden said that Mentoring in Medicine discusses racism from the beginning, and that their school-based programs incorporate a segment on health care disparities. For older students in undergraduate and postbaccalaureate programs, Mentoring in Medicine has speakers and mentors who discuss the challenges they have faced in their education and careers. The program also has psychiatrists and psychologists who discuss what racism is and strategies to deal with racist acts as well as the psychological stress of racism. Lanier responded that, "At the community college, I think the students kind of already know that coming in the door, that there is something going on relative to race." Nevertheless, he emphasized the importance of Black leaders and physicians affirming these students' experiences of racism. Moreover, he suggested that hearing about the challenges experienced by those who have achieved academic and professional success, such as the leaders in the room, would "affirm and seal and strengthen" the ability of these students to persevere. Finally, he suggested the need to support students in navigating their experiences of racism, provide strategies they can employ to maintain

---

[10] Owen is dean and chancellor of Ross University School of Medicine.

[11] Hurley is professor of medicine and orthopedics and associate dean at UConn Health.

[12] Laurencin is university professor, Van Dusen Distinguished Professor of Orthopaedic Surgery, and director, The Raymond and Beverly Sackler Center at the University of Connecticut.

[13] Bright is associate dean for Inclusive Excellence, director of the Office of Special Programs, and associate professor of medicine at the University of North Carolina School of Medicine.

their mental health in the face of racism and discrimination, and advocate for students. Britt expanded on Lanier's last comment, describing the need for better encouragement and advisement from mentors and counselors, especially when students are met with challenges and barriers. Whereas other students may be encouraged to persist and to try again if they encounter barriers or failures, Black boys and men may not receive the same encouragement to overcome these challenges.

REFERENCES

Holden, L., B. Rumala, P. Carson, and E. Siegel. 2014. Promoting careers in health care for urban youth: What students, parents and educators can teach us. *Information Services and Use* 34(3–4):355–366. https://www.ncbi.nlm.nih.gov/pmc/articles/PMC4286884 (accessed February 26, 2018).

Skiba, R. J., R. S. Michael, A. C. Nardo, and R. Peterson. 2000. The color of discipline: Sources of racial and gender disproportionality in school punishment. Bloomington, IN: Indiana Education Policy Center. https://eric.ed.gov/?id=ED468512 (accessed May 4, 2018).

Skiba, R. J., R. H. Horner, C.-G. Chung, M. K. Rausch, S. L. May, and T. Tobin. 2011. Race is not neutral: A national investigation of African American and Latino disproportionality in school discipline. *School Psychology Review* 40(1):85–107. https://search.proquest.com/openview/a7389dd1667724ca0e8dd8102f1a107c/1?pq-origsite=gscholar&cbl=48217 (accessed May 4, 2018).

Wallace, J. M., S. Goodkind, C. M. Wallace, and J. G. Bachman. 2008. Racial, ethnic, and gender differences in school discipline among U.S. high school students: 1991–2005. *Negro Educational Review* 59(1–2):47–62. https://www.ncbi.nlm.nih.gov/pmc/articles/PMC2678799 (accessed May 4, 2018).

5

Current Innovative and Exploratory Strategies to Support Entry into Science and Medicine for Black Men

Highlights Presented by Individual Speakers

- Focusing solely on low-income students may miss capturing Black students of higher socioeconomic position who still underperform and are underrepresented relative to peers of other racial and ethnic backgrounds, and especially compared with White peers. (Moore)
- Interventions to address barriers to advancement along the educational pipeline are needed at multiple transition points (for example, between middle school and high school, high school and college). (Reede)
- Commitment from faculty and leadership, applying evidence and data, and building cohorts supported by mentors are key elements of successful pipeline programs. (Hrabowski)
- Leadership's belief that pipeline programs are important and committing financial resources were key to successfully implementing the Vanderbilt University School of Medicine African American and Disadvantaged Student Pipeline Program. (Churchwell)
- Focusing on Black boys should not reduce efforts that have led to advances and achievements among Black girls. (Powell, Reede)

- Undergraduate students are "low hanging fruit" on whom pipeline interventions should focus in the near terms (next few years), because this pool of students could become competitive in health professions admission with relatively little support and additional preparation. (Hrabowski)
- Structural interventions should complement individual-focused pipeline programs. (Jones)
- Barriers to structural thinking include focusing on the individual, ahistorical thinking, and the myth of meritocracy. (Jones)

This panel focused on current programs to strengthen the medical educational pipeline through greater support of underrepresented minority students, and especially Black boys and men. André L. Churchwell, M.D.,[1] presented a pipeline program for undergraduate students at Vanderbilt University. James L. Moore III, Ph.D.,[2] discussed lessons learned from work at the Todd A. Bell National Resource Center on the African American Male at The Ohio State University. Marja Hurley, M.D.,[3] described a range of pipeline programs at UConn Health. Joan Y. Reede, M.D., M.S., M.P.H., M.B.A.,[4] described pipeline programs and lessons learned at Harvard Medical School. Freeman Hrabowski III, Ph.D.,[5] moderated the session and led a brief discussion following the presentations.

MEYERHOFF SCHOLARS PROGRAM

Freeman Hrabowski III, Ph.D.
President
University of Maryland, Baltimore County

To launch the discussion, Hrabowski briefly described the Meyerhoff Scholars Program at the UMBC,[6] which provides financial support, men-

---

[1] Churchwell is Levi Watkins, Jr., M.D. chair and chief diversity officer at the Vanderbilt University Medical Center and senior associate dean for diversity affairs at the Vanderbilt University School of Medicine.

[2] Moore is interim vice provost for diversity and inclusion and chief diversity officer, executive director of the Todd A. Bell National Resource Center on the African American Male, and College of Education and Human Ecology distinguished professor of urban education at The Ohio State University.

[3] Hurley is professor of medicine and orthopedics at the University of Connecticut (UConn) School of Medicine and associate dean for the Health Career Opportunity Programs at UConn Health.

[4] Reede is dean for diversity and community partnership at Harvard Medical School.

[5] Hrabowski is president of the University of Maryland, Baltimore County (UMBC).

[6] For more information about the Meyerhoff Scholars Program, see https://meyerhoff.umbc.edu (accessed February 28, 2018).

toring and advising, and exposure to research to undergraduate students committed to increasing the representation of minorities in science and engineering and to obtaining Ph.D. degrees in math, science, and engineering.[7] He commented on the program's successes, noting that UMBC is the top producer of African American M.D./Ph.D. recipients, having produced 42 M.D./Ph.D.s since 2000, with relative parity among men and women. From his experience with the Meyerhoff program, Hrabowski identified key elements necessary for successful pipeline programs. First, he emphasized the importance of a school's commitment to increasing the number of African American science graduates. He remarked, "If we really want to see a difference . . . the culture of the institution has to change. It has to be a priority." He elaborated that both faculty and leadership, including top administrative staff like university presidents and deans, are crucial to driving change. Second, he noted the importance of applying evidence and data, saying "We are much too warm and fuzzy when talking about these issues. We need to focus on having a culture that will emphasize analytics and look at who succeeds and what it takes to succeed." Finally, Hrabowski underscored the importance of building cohorts that collaborate, support each other, and are accountable to each other, and which are also supported by mentors.

VANDERBILT UNIVERSITY SCHOOL OF MEDICINE AFRICAN AMERICAN AND DISADVANTAGED STUDENT PIPELINE PROGRAM

André L. Churchwell, M.D.
Levi Watkins Jr., M.D. Chair and Chief Diversity Officer
Vanderbilt University Medical Center
Professor of Medicine (Cardiology), Professor of Radiology and Radiological Sciences, Professor of Biomedical Engineering, and Senior Associate Dean for Diversity Affairs
Vanderbilt University School of Medicine

The Vanderbilt University School of Medicine (VUSM) recently implemented a "short pipeline" program. The program is a partnership among three Historically Black Colleges and Universities (HBCUs)—Morehouse College, Spelman College, and Fisk University. The fourth institution included in the partnership, Berea College, has a long history of provid-

[7] The first cohort of Meyerhoff Scholars comprised 19 African American men. The second cohort expanded to include African American women, and in 1996, the program was opened to students of all backgrounds. For the 2017–2018 academic year, 260 students enrolled in the program, of whom 63 percent identify as African American, 15 percent as Caucasian, 11 percent as Asian, 10 percent as Hispanic, and 1 percent as Native American.

ing undergraduate education for minority and international students. The program is designed to support underrepresented minorities who intend to pursue medical education, which provides a direct path for admission to VUSM. The program applies holistic criteria to select undergraduate premedical students. The program then connects selected students with faculty and current medical student mentors and provides tutoring and academic support throughout their 4 years. Students also participate in a summer program that includes coursework in the basic sciences, Medical College Admission Test (MCAT) preparation, and research experiences. Students are provisionally admitted to VUSM and those who maintain a grade point average and achieve MCAT scores that have been jointly agreed upon by the undergraduate schools and VUSM matriculate into VUSM. The first cohort of four rising college sophomores was inducted in the summer of 2017.[8] As a lesson for other schools that intend to replicate or scale this type of program, Churchwell identified commitment from leadership, including both the belief that the program is important, and the commitment of financial resources, as key to the program's successful implementation. He added,

> The goal here is to try to create some type of connection. . . . [We] believe that this is an important thing to do, number one. Number two, the students feel warm and fuzzy, and they are connected to us. Three, we try to diminish the idea of [applying for and matriculating to medical school] being just an insurmountable hurdle by going through the selection process and giving them the premed curriculum and a lot of tests along the way to generate their confidence to build their idea of success of coming into [VUSM].

Churchwell also presented his Marshall Plan for American education, a proposal to create a national pipeline program to support a broader range of underrepresented minorities and disadvantaged groups. In this program, Churchwell envisions schools of the Association of American Universities as statewide hubs, supported by a national superstructure that is connected to the federal government. These hubs would be connected to HBCUs and other colleges, K–12 school systems, state and national educational departments and leadership, education experts, and philanthropic organizations, among others. See Figure 5-1 for more detail.

[8] For more information on the VUSM "short pipeline" program, see https://news.vanderbilt.edu/2017/07/27/school-of-medicine-programs-enhancing-diversity-of-applicants (accessed February 28, 2018).

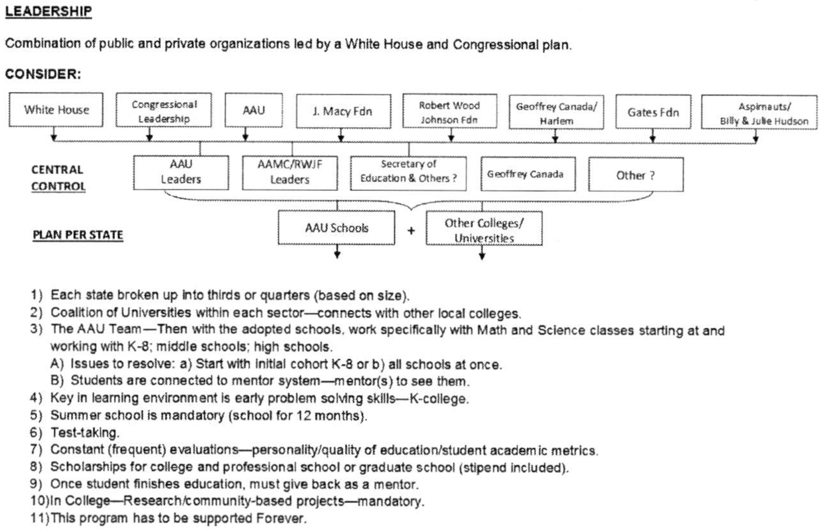

FIGURE 5-1 The Marshall Plan for American education.
NOTE: AAMC = Association of American Medical Colleges; AAU = Association of American Universities; Fdn = Foundation; J. Macy Fdn = The Josiah Macy Jr. Foundation; K = kindergarten; RWJF = Robert Wood Johnson Foundation.
SOURCE: Presentation by André L. Churchwell, November 20, 2018.

THE OHIO STATE UNIVERSITY BELL NATIONAL RESOURCE CENTER ON THE AFRICAN AMERICAN MALE

James L. Moore III, Ph.D.
Interim Vice Provost for Diversity and Inclusion and Chief Diversity Officer
Executive Director, Todd A. Bell National Resource Center on the African American Male
College of Education and Human Ecology
Distinguished Professor of Urban Education
The Ohio State University

Moore began his presentation by highlighting the need to focus on racial disparities and not just socioeconomic status. He reasoned that, although race and socioeconomic status are correlated, focusing solely on low-income students may miss capturing Black students of higher socioeconomic position who still underperform and are underrepresented relative to peers of other racial and ethnic backgrounds, and especially compared with White peers. Moore next described what he called his "ethos of excellence," which states that attaining achievements (e.g., educational and professional attainment) is the product of competence (or skills), and confidence (or will). Focusing on the latter, he distinguished between persistence and resilience. He commented, "Persistence is the constant sustained effort. Resilience is bouncing back. How do we help young people—you don't even have to motivate them; they get up just on their own and they do their work on their own." Moore also identified several psychological barriers that can discourage Black men from pursuing medical and science careers. These include "invisibility syndrome,"[9] an emotional response to discrimination and racism "when [a student's] sense of humanity has not been affirmed," and the minority tax,[10] or additional responsibilities placed on minorities and the expectation that these minorities represent their otherness across an institution, among others.

Moore briefly discussed the history and mission of the Bell National Resource Center on the African American Male[11] at The Ohio State University, which examines and addresses issues pertaining to African American males throughout the life span. The center conducts research and produces reports on and identifies best practices regarding African American men, and serves as a resource on African American men for government agencies and colleges and universities across the country. The center also supports and fosters community among African American men at The Ohio State University, offering professional development, counseling, and positive reinforcement for achieving academic goals, as well as connecting students to research experiences, scholarships, and other opportunities.

From the center's research, Moore identified five factors that influence the life and career development of African American men: interests, preparation, experiences, connections, and opportunity. In terms of interests, he commented that although they know how to get people interested in science, technology, engineering, and mathematics (STEM), less is known about how to sustain these interests. With regard to preparation, he emphasized that, although many discussions focus on K–12 education, preparation is needed throughout the educational pipeline. Experiences refer to the need to ensure that students "have experiences

[9] For more information on invisibility syndrome, see https://www.ncbi.nlm.nih.gov/pubmed/10702848 (accessed February 28, 2018).

[10] For more information on the minority tax, see Darrell Kirch's presentation in Chapter 2. Also see https://bmcmededuc.biomedcentral.com/articles/10.1186/s12909-015-0290-9 (accessed February 21, 2018) and https://jamanetwork.com/journals/jama/fullarticle/2625322 (accessed February 21, 2018).

[11] For more information on the Bell National Resource Center on the African American Male, see https://odi.osu.edu/bell-national-resource-center (accessed April 30, 2018).

that are indicative to the spaces in which they are expected to work." Connections pertain primarily to connecting students to mentors. Finally, regarding opportunity, Moore described the need to not only offer opportunities to African American male students, but also to get them to take opportunities when offered.

AETNA HEALTH PROFESSIONS PARTNERSHIP INITIATIVE (HPPI) SCHOLARS DOCTORS PIPELINE

Marja Hurley, M.D.
Professor of Medicine and Orthopedics, UConn School of Medicine
Associate Dean for Health Career Opportunity Programs, UConn Health

The Department of Health Career Opportunity Programs at UConn Health administers the Aetna Health Professions Partnership Initiative (HPPI) Scholars Doctors Pipeline, a continuous pipeline of programs for students in middle school through college, as well as their parents (see Figure 5-2).[12] The pipeline program seeks to develop the pool of underrepresented minority applicants to health professional schools, primarily at UConn. For the middle school and high school programs, the program partners with two public school systems, the New Britain and Hartford public school systems; for the undergraduate programs, it partners with local universities, including the UConn campuses in Storrs and Hartford, Connecticut, and Central Connecticut State University. These programs include science and nonscience academic enrichment, college and test preparation, exposure to STEM careers (e.g., clinical shadowing), research experience, mentoring, professional development, and opportunities for presentation. The Department of Health Career Opportunity Programs promotes an academically and socially supportive environment for those students who matriculate to UConn health professional schools.

Hurley provided select program outcomes. The Senior Doctors Academy offers year-round enrichment and, for qualified students, an earned stipend to high school seniors who are interested in medicine, dental medicine, or biomedical research, and who come from low-income families and/or are in the first generation in their families to attend college.[13] Of 171 participants, 5 are currently enrolled in the UConn School of

---

[12] For more information on the Aetna Health Professions Partnership Initiative (HPPI) Scholars Doctors Pipeline programs at UConn Health, see https://health.uconn.edu/hcop (accessed February 28, 2018).

[13] For more information on the Senior Doctors Academy, see https://health.uconn.edu/hcop/enrichment-programs/senior-doctors-academy (accessed March 16, 2018).

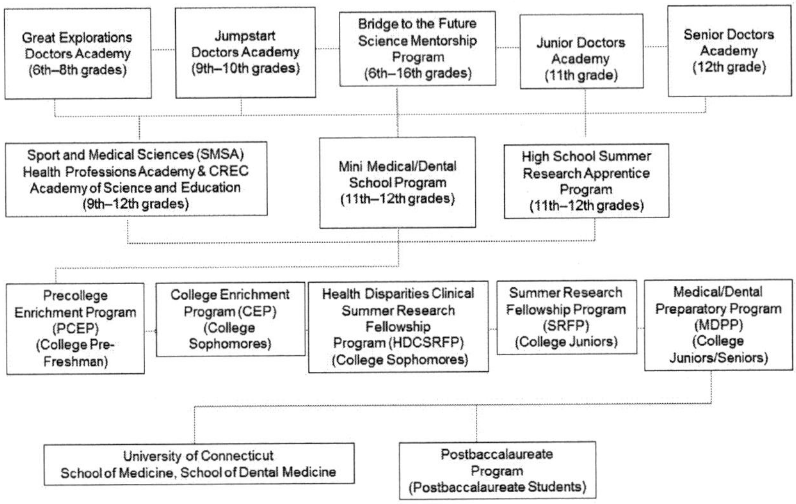

FIGURE 5-2 UConn Health Aetna Health Professions Partnership Initiative (HPPI) Scholars Doctors Pipeline.
SOURCE: Presentation by Marja Hurley, November 20, 2018.

Medicine, 4 entered pharmacy school, 3 are in nursing, 6 are pursuing allied health professions, 1 is pursuing biomedical research, 1 is enrolled in dental school, and 3 are enrolled in postbaccalaureate programs. There are 70 students still enrolled in undergraduate studies, and 46 students pursued nonhealth professions. Outcomes for 31 are unknown, which includes participants who moved out of the target school districts or who withdrew or were otherwise dismissed from the program. One student is deceased. Hurley commented that sustaining program commitment for all 4 years of high school, especially among Black and Hispanic male students, is challenging.

The Health Disparities Clinical Summer Research Fellowship Program places rising college sophomores, juniors, and seniors or recent college graduates in community health centers or other organizations working with underserved populations.[14] The program also requires participants to develop and present a research program related to health disparities. Of 103 participants, 31 entered medical school, 11 entered dental school, 19 entered other health professional schools (e.g., nursing, allied

[14] For more information on the Health Disparities Clinical Summer Research Fellowship Program, see https://health.uconn.edu/hcop/enrichment-programs/health-disparities-clinical-summer-research-fellowship-program (accessed March 16, 2018).

health, pharmacy), 2 are enrolled in graduate programs, 7 decided they were not interested in health careers, and 33 students are still completing their undergraduate degrees. The Medical and Dental Preparatory Program and Summer Research Fellowship Program place undergraduates in a biomedical research lab and provide opportunities for clinical shadowing and presentation. Of 823 program participants from 1996 to 2017, 658 entered the health professions—349 went to medical school, 161 to dental school, 40 to graduate schools, and 109 to other health professions; 39 program graduates pursued careers not in the health professions, and 60 are still undergraduates. Overall, of 195 African American and Hispanic students who graduated from the UConn School of Medicine from 2003 to 2017, 80 participated in HPPI pipeline programs; of 84 African American and Hispanic students who graduated from the UConn School of Dentistry in the same period, 40 participated in pipeline programs.

HARVARD MEDICAL SCHOOL OFFICE FOR DIVERSITY, INCLUSION, AND COMMUNITY PARTNERSHIP

Joan Y. Reede, M.D.
Dean for Diversity and Community Partnership
Harvard Medical School

Reede started her presentation by pointing out,

> We talk about this as though there are these children in the mental health system and children in the educational system and children in our clinics. We are talking about the same children. And when we think of solutions we need to think beyond those of us who are in the health professions; we need to think beyond those in the academy, and [think about] how do our communities come together to support our youth.
>
> I think about our children as swimming upstream, going to schools where they are unprepared, where the schools do not have quality education, or sometimes the resources they need, where they don't have the mentors, they don't have the role models, they don't have the opportunities, but we are telling them to survive.
>
> Oftentimes when we talk about health disparities, we talk about the social determinants of health. Those same social determinants of health are impacting the youth that we're talking about, and you cannot separate it. Those same issues of if you are hungry, if you don't have a place to sleep, if you don't feel safe, they impact your learning.

In addition to these social factors, Reede also identified racism, discrimination, and bias, and resulting effects such as stereotype threat, microaggressions, lack of validation, isolation and exclusion, tokenism, and "being hypervisible and invisible at the same time" as barriers to these students' success. She elaborated on the need to address these barriers to advancement throughout the educational pipeline at each of the junctures at which students might enter, exit, and re-enter the pipeline along the multiple paths students might follow.

Reede then described the pipeline programs of the Office for Diversity, Inclusion, and Community Partnerships at Harvard Medical School, themes across the programs, and lessons learned. Harvard programs include educational outreach to K–12 students, the Biomedical Science Careers Program, and The Commonwealth Fund Mongan Fellowships in Minority Health Policy. The educational outreach K–12 programs include in-school programming—developing curricula used in schools, teacher professional development, and working with the College Board to help teachers to teach advanced placement courses—and out-of-school programming for middle and high school students, and college students both during the academic year and during summer breaks.[15]

The Biomedical Science Careers Program is a partnership between internal Harvard individuals, offices, departments, and institutions, and external partners from industry (e.g., biotechnology, pharmaceutical, and medical device companies), law firms, medical schools, community colleges, and community organizations that produces conferences and symposiums. The program offers scholarships, workshops, mentoring and advising, and other resources to support students from high school through postdoctoral fellowships who wish to pursue biomedical careers. Since it was established in 1991, roughly 13,000 students, residents, and fellows have participated in the program.[16] The Commonwealth Fund Mongan Fellowship is a 1-year fellowship for physicians committed to transforming health care delivery systems for vulnerable populations and is a "deliberate effort to create leaders who could create change." Fellows complete coursework leading to a master of public health or a master of public administration degree at Harvard and participate in forums and seminars with leaders in health care delivery, public policy, and minority health.[17]

Reede identified the following themes across the Harvard Medical School pipeline programs: continuity, consistency, collaboration, creativ-

[15] For more information on the Harvard Medical School Office of Diversity, Inclusion, and Community Partnerships programs, see https://mfdp.med.harvard.edu (accessed March 2, 2018).

[16] For more information on the Biomedical Science Careers Program, see http://www.bscp.org (accessed March 2, 2018).

[17] For more information on the Commonwealth Fund Mongan Fellowship in Minority Health, see http://www.commonwealthfund.org/grants-and-fellowships/fellowships/commonwealth-fund-mongan-fellowship-in-minority-health-policy (accessed March 2, 2018) and https://mfdp.med.harvard.edu/cfmf (accessed March 2, 2018).

ity, communication, consideration, and commitment. Continuity refers to continuity of efforts across academic levels, or, ensuring linkages when students bridge different educational levels (e.g., middle to high school). Consistency refers to consistent efforts over time, and not funding or implementing programs for only a few years at a time. Collaboration means not being territorial or competitive across different health professions, allowing students to choose the health career path they desire, and not expecting them to follow the choices made for them. This also includes collaboration across institutions to create a system to support students, not only within their individual schools and universities, but across schools as well. Creativity describes the capacity to be innovative in developing new programs and "not doing the same things that we have always done that did not work." Communication pertains to communicating with students and meeting them where they are, on the platforms they are using, and not only through traditional academic channels. Consideration refers to recognition and acknowledgment of intersectionality, and people's multiple identities. Reede commented, "There are all sorts of ways people are in the margins, and we have multiple identities" and queried how academic leaders can recognize those identities. Finally, Reede pointed out the need to identify ways to stay committed to these initiatives and this goal, as well as how to get leadership engaged and committed.

Reede closed her presentation with the following lessons learned from implementing pipeline programs:

- Set an explicit goal or sets of goals.
- Set a realistic time frame.
- Put forward a rationale for the program, and align it with the organization's mission.
- Assess data and evaluate programs to build an evidence base of effective programs.
- Have a seamless articulation of programs.
- Create opportunities for multiple points of entry, exit, and re-entry.
- Be flexible and adjust to environmental and policy changes and to local needs.
- Engage communities.
- Cross boundaries and disciplines.
- Think in terms of multilevel and dynamic systems and connections across systems.
- Provide not just academic but also career development.
- Track, monitor, and evaluate for continuous improvement.

DISCUSSION

Wizdom Powell, Ph.D.,[18] commented that the discussions of pipeline interventions to increase representation of Black boys in medical education often assume a zero-sum proposition between Black boys and Black girls—or, that increasing focus on boys and men should decrease focus on women and girls. However, she offered that this need not be the case—a focus on Black boys should not reduce efforts that have successfully led to advances and achievements among Black girls. Hrabowski expanded on these comments, saying,

> We sometimes end up pitting one group against another, [but] we should be celebrating the success that some African Americans have had . . . it's the genius of the "and" versus the tyranny of the "or." We have to keep lifting women up, celebrating what they are doing, and get them to help us push more men to do well.

Reede concurred with Powell and cautioned against inflating the successes of Black girls and women. Despite their advances, she suggested that there is still room for improvement, saying,

> I do think this idea of pitting men against women and Black men against Black women makes no kind of sense whatsoever. As we talk about Black women doing better, there are roughly 145 medical schools. There are 180 Black female full professors across [these schools], so there are only like one per medical school, and there are 12 Black female chairs. That doesn't mean that this is not a critically important issue around our Black men, but we should make sure that we don't depict this as though the Black women have reached nirvana, because they have not.

Camara Jones, M.D., M.P.H., Ph.D.,[19] emphasized the need for structural interventions to even the playing field, which complement the individual-focused pipeline programs. She cautioned,

> When we do not name those systems of structured inequity, when we do not say even the word racism, we are complicit with the widespread denial that racism continues to exist. When we don't talk about those systems and try to address those, when people see that there are uneven outcomes, they blame this one [child] instead of thinking these are chil-

[18] Powell is director of the Health Disparities Institute and associate professor of psychiatry at UConn Health.

[19] Jones is senior fellow at the Satcher Health Leadership Institute at Morehouse School of Medicine.

> dren with equal potential and they had different circumstances. They say this one was lazy or stupid. And we are all buying into that.

Jones identified three barriers to structural thinking. She said,

> There are three huge barriers in this country that we are going to face no matter what we try to do to set it right. The first is this narrow focus on the individual that makes systems and structures either appear to be invisible or irrelevant, and it also makes us feel like what can I do as opposed to what can we do as a collective. The second is that we as a nation are ahistorical, and we act as if the current distribution of resources, advantaged, disadvantaged, is just a happenstance, and we act as if the present is disconnected from the past. The third is this myth of meritocracy. The story goes something like this. If you work hard, you will make it. . . . Now, most people who have made it have worked hard, but there are many others who are working just as hard or harder who will never make it because of this uneven playing field—racism, sexism, heterosexist, all those things that are structured and are perpetuating the uneven playing field.

Hrabowski wrapped up the discussion by identifying the important points made by the panel, in his opinion. First, he identified the need for data, analytics, and rigorous analysis to know which of these pipeline programs and which elements of these programs work. Second, he proposed a focus on undergraduate students in the near term (next few years) as "low hanging fruit." He commented that there are undergraduate students who are interested in STEM careers, but face challenges, such as a bad grade in a science or math course early in their undergraduate careers, and this experience often discourages them from continuing their pursuit of STEM. Thus, he suggested that this pool of students could become competitive in health professions admission with relatively little support and additional preparation. Finally, he described the need to think more creatively about academic preparation, not restricting undergraduate students who wish to pursue health professions to science majors, and strengthening academic preparation through nonscience coursework.

6

Reflections on Meeting Day 1

Highlights Presented by Individual Speakers

- The shortage of Black men in medicine is not an intractable problem, but it is hard, because institutional racism is a fundamental barrier. (Prothrow-Stith)
- Political advocacy and action are needed to address the culture of schools where structures of institutional racism disadvantage students at an early age and have lifelong effects. (Mallett)
- A national clearinghouse of pipeline programs can offer those interested in implementing programs a resource to identify effective programs with attributes that match their community and its needs, connections to the individuals running these programs, and support for program design and implementation. (Montgomery Rice)
- Identifying priority issues, developing a strategy to address the issue that incorporates measurable outcomes, and setting a timeline are critical for moving forward. (Montgomery Rice)
- Building cohorts, cultivating interest in science, technology, engineering, and mathematics (STEM) from a young age, and helping students to manage financial circumstances are key strategies to encourage students to pursue STEM careers. (Frederick)

In the final session on the first day of the meeting, leadership from four Historically Black Colleges and Universities (HBCUs) offered reflections on the barriers for Black men's entry to medicine and current strategies to address these challenges. The panelists were Valerie Montgomery Rice, M.D.; Wayne A. I. Frederick, M.D., M.B.A., FACS; Veronica Mallett, M.D., M.M.M.; and Deborah Prothrow-Stith, M.D.[1] L. D. Britt, M.D.,[2] moderated a brief open audience discussion following the panel. The first day of the workshop closed with a poster session presenting perspectives from current medical students.

REFLECTIONS

Valerie Montgomery Rice, M.D.
President and Dean
Morehouse School of Medicine

Montgomery Rice reflected on the medical educational pipeline and the junctures at which boys are lost. Using the analogy of a leaky pipeline she developed, she reviewed the number of African American boys and men who

- do not complete high school;
- graduate but do not enroll in college;
- do not matriculate to or complete college;
- apply or take the Medical College Admission Test (MCAT) in preparation for medical school, but do not apply to medical school or do not get accepted; and
- become physicians.

She also touched on high rates of incarceration, family structure, and low socioeconomic status as some social and environmental factors that may influence the low achievement rates.

Montgomery Rice then presented the idea of a national clearinghouse for pipeline programs, a proposal for which is included in the Morehouse School of Medicine's strategic plan. It would be a database of pipeline programs like those discussed over the course of the day, a resource to share what works. The clearinghouse would also require programs to

[1] Montgomery Rice is president and dean of the Morehouse School of Medicine; Frederick is president of Howard University; Mallett is dean of the School of Medicine at Meharry Medical College; and Prothrow-Stith is dean and professor of medicine for the College of Medicine at the Charles R. Drew University.

[2] Britt is Henry Ford professor and Edward J. Brickhouse chairman of the Department of Surgery at Eastern Virginia Medical School.

have specific objectives and would use standardized metrics to assess program outcomes. Those looking to implement a program could search the clearinghouse for programs with attributes that match their community and its needs. Recognizing the importance of flexible programs with the capacity to adapt and be responsive to local environments, Montgomery Rice commented that the clearinghouse would offer a start, connections to those running successful programs, and development and implementation support.

Next, Montgomery Rice discussed the problem of declining African American applicants and matriculants to HBCU medical schools since 2002. The deans of the four HBCU medical schools represented on the panel—Charles R. Drew University of Medicine and Science, Howard University, Meharry Medical College, and the Morehouse School of Medicine—convened the Empower Conference, an annual conference launched in 2016, which seeks to address the decline of African American students from HBCUs who pursue health and science.[3] For the 2018 conference, some workshops will address strengthening undergraduate curriculum, MCAT preparation, and financial and social determinants.

Montgomery Rice closed her presentation with a call to action. She declared,

> We need to walk away from here with a plan to work on one of these issues or two of these issues, three of these issues, and we need to have a strategy that is marked by expected outcomes. We have to have a timeline, and we have to be able to measure it. And finally, what you do matters every day. . . . Being present matters.

Wayne A. I. Frederick, M.D., M.B.A., FACS
President
Howard University

Frederick first briefly described how Howard University is working to increase the applicant pool and number of African American students from HBCUs in its medical school. For 3 years, select undergraduate students from HBCUs are invited to come to Howard for medical school for the summer to receive didactic instruction and MCAT/test preparation, with paid accommodations. Since implementing the program, the number of HBCUs represented in the freshman medical school has risen from five (including Howard) to nine (also including Howard). He commented on the need to increase opportunity within HBCUs, saying,

---

[3] For more information, see http://empowerconf.com/Support_Files/HBCUEmpowerCommissionedPaper.pdf (accessed March 5, 2018).

> I think it's extremely important that we first extend ourselves to our fellow HBCUs in terms of pipelining. There is a great opportunity there. There are lots of students who are interested, but especially because of the fact that they may not have professional programs on their campuses or access to some of the prep programs that are necessary, we have to ensure that we are giving them an opportunity to do so.

Frederick also described a new science, technology, engineering, and mathematics (STEM) Scholar Program at Howard, which supports undergraduates interested in pursuing a Ph.D. or M.D./Ph.D. in a STEM field.[4] He remarked that for these high-achieving students, many had competing offers from Ivy League schools, but chose Howard because they valued participation in a cohort.

Frederick discussed lessons learned from the Howard experience. First, he commented on the importance of community and cultivating supportive but also accountable environments. He said,

> I think we have an environment at our schools where these types of students can thrive, and certainly we can provide the right types of opportunities in order to make sure that they are interested. . . . Howard, at orientation, one of the conversations that people were subjected to is that you would look to your left and look to your right and the people there would not be there. . . . What I encourage the students to remember is that the person to the left and the person to the right needs to be at graduation with you. So, you have a responsibility to the community around you to make sure that everyone is getting there.

Frederick described the need to identify and cultivate interests. He described the need to expose young Black boys to STEM in middle school, encourage undergraduate students with interest and competences to pursue STEM careers, and support students' interest with better advising at the undergraduate level starting in the freshman year. To increase retention and graduation rates, Howard has increased opportunities for STEM undergraduates. For example, Howard has a program for biology majors to pick a track within biology that provides opportunities for research and for exposure in hospitals. Howard's Office of Undergraduate Studies also helps address financial barriers, helping to manage students' financial circumstances and offering a 50 percent tuition rebate for direct tuition payments for the final semester for students who graduate on time.

[4] For more information on the STEM Scholars Program at Howard University, see https://www2.howard.edu/scholarships/bison-stem-scholars (accessed April 11, 2018).

Veronica Mallett, M.D., M.M.M.
Dean, School of Medicine
Meharry Medical College

Mallett reflected on disparities in the public education system and how they contribute to the dearth of Black men in medicine. She commented that, on one end of the spectrum, some Black boys in some underresourced schools in low-income neighborhoods are ostracized, stereotyped, and their behavior criminalized. On the other end, some high-performing schools have supportive environments and produce exceptional students. Mallett noted that this disadvantage has consequences throughout the life span, saying, "A growing number of students start kindergarten already trailing their privileged counterparts, and they rarely if ever catch up." She added that these disparities are not incidental, but instead result from institutional racism and specific actions such as privileged people paying and lobbying for better schools and better resources in schools. Given that this racist educational infrastructure results from specific actions, it is neither inexorable nor unalterable. Mallett said, "We can do something about that, and we can hold the public school system accountable." Specifically, she endorsed political advocacy and action to change the culture of schools and to address the institutional racism that structures disadvantage for students at an early age and has lifelong effects. "We really need to focus on healing the culture in public schools," she said.

Deborah Prothrow-Stith, M.D.
Dean, College of Medicine
Charles R. Drew University

Prothrow-Stith discussed her list of significant points from the day's panels and discussions. She opened her comments by acknowledging the role of HBCUs in providing supportive environments and cohorts. She said,

> A house that is built for you is very different from a house in which you are invited as a guest. Not all of us are in need of a house built for us, but that is what the HBCUs sort of bring to this table, and I think it is really important to recognize.

Prothrow-Stith then noted that the shortage of Black men in medicine is not an intractable problem. She said, "It's not rocket science. We know what is needed. But it is hard because . . . it's institutional racism that we are up against." She then listed the following strategies as potential ways to address the problem:

- Changing public policy,
- Supporting and growing existing programs,
- Starting early and providing continuous support for students,
- Naming racism,
- Creating role models to change norms (i.e., negative public perceptions and images) about Black men and increase the career attractiveness of medicine and other STEM careers for Black men, and
- Addressing financial barriers.

DISCUSSION

To launch the discussion, moderator Britt posed two questions for the panelists. First, he asked what specific strategies they would implement if given $20 billion, or $2 billion every year for 10 years. Montgomery Rice started by saying she would do the following:

- Centralize and create a clearinghouse of pipeline programs such that any community would be able to apply for receiving funding for pipeline programs.
- Start a new medical school committed to diversity and inclusion.
- Partner with four major health systems to advance the residency training opportunities.

Frederick said he would do the following:

- Create a network of middle and high schools around existing HBCUs.
- Create a network of HBCUs and medical schools that have a focus on diversity.
- Focus on interprofessional education between medicine and other health professions.

Mallett would do the following:

- Create a moratorium on out-of-school suspensions and use restorative approaches to discipline in public schools.
- Foster a curriculum rebirth in HBCUs and, echoing Frederick, create a network of HBCU and diversity-focused medical schools.
- Foster campus partnerships with Greek organizations and service organizations to promote positive attitudes about excellence in learning and educational attainment.
- Create a task force to look at other educational systems and identify lessons from international experience.

Next, Britt asked the panelists what outcome measures should be used to evaluate the efficacy of the strategies implemented. Frederick said health care disparities, Prothrow-Stith offered metrics throughout the educational system, and Reede put forward a metric for systems change. Reede also proposed training researchers to develop new methodologies and metrics beyond standard ways of thinking about measuring advancement and success.

General Discussion

Montgomery Rice discussed the need for partnerships with "unlikely bedfellows." She gave the example of insurers and suggested they might be good partners because they already collect and maintain a lot of data such as demographic information (including on race and ethnicity and other social factors) and health- and disease-related information, and because they can enroll their members in trials to test the efficacy and efficiency of programs.

Arthur C. Evans, Jr., Ph.D.,[5] proposed taking a life span developmental perspective to move forward. He described a need to think holistically about challenges and barriers throughout the medical education pipeline in order to best address them. He remarked,

> You just cannot take one part of the pipeline . . . to deal with this issue. . . . We may want to think about what are the dimensions across that life span developmental perspective and how do those issues change depending on the developmental milestones that young men and boys are dealing with.

Evans also discussed using this life span perspective to examine the efficacy and efficiency of pipeline programs over time. He closed by suggesting the need to build and work with allies—to engage mentors and leaders who are not African American who can nevertheless support and provide insights into ways to increase the representation of Black men in medicine.

POSTER SESSION: INNOVATIVE APPROACHES TO BLACK MEN IN MEDICINE (STUDENT PERSPECTIVES)

The first day of the workshop closed with a poster session in which medical students offered their perspectives. Ross McMillan and Robert Wardlow, M.D./Ph.D. candidates from the Johns Hopkins School of

---

[5] Evans is chief executive officer of the American Psychological Association.

Medicine, and Gabriel Felix, a 3rd-year medical student at Howard University College of Medicine, presented "The Need for More of Us: Perspectives and Solutions for Increasing Black Men in Medicine by Black Men in Medicine." Abbas Rattani, M.Be., a 3rd-year medical student at Loyola University Chicago Stritch School of Medicine, presented "Improving Black Male Matriculation in Medicine through Fashion as Art and Activism." Martin Campbell, a 2nd-year medical student at Morehouse School of Medicine, presented "Black Men in Medicine: A Novel Approach to Mentorship and Policy Reform."

7

Accountability in Medicine: What Can Medical Schools Do to Address the Crisis?

Highlights Presented by Individual Speakers

- The quality of mentors is important. Mentoring and tailoring learning to students' needs, including different learning styles, are important to ensure students' success. Programs to guide interested mentors in how best to do so can help to ensure that well-intentioned mentors do not inadvertently harm their mentees. (Azar, Carson)
- Addressing social determinants such as housing and residential environments can help students to succeed. (Carson)
- To better understand differences in educational performance among Black students, disaggregating data on U.S.- and foreign-born Black students is needed. The educational achievement and health disparities experienced by native-born Blacks that result from a legacy of disadvantage and discrimination in the United States may not be comparable to the educational and sociocultural experiences of foreign-born Blacks, which, in some cases, may reflect privilege. (Wilson)
- The highly diverse student body at the University of Illinois College of Medicine is attributable to the school's faculty, a commitment to diversity, a focus on excellence, the efforts of associate deans for diversity and inclusion, and an emphasis on the value of education. (Azar)

- Efforts to attract, train, and retain underrepresented minorities in medicine and other sectors will require systems thinking, culturally based solutions, individual encouragement and strong role models, and grassroots efforts. (Azar)
- New technologies may offer potential solutions for addressing the challenge of the absence of Black men in medicine. (Azar)
- Including diversity goals as key performance indicators for leadership ensure accountability for diversity at Ross University School of Medicine. Having accountability at the level of leadership removes the responsibility for increasing diversity at the level of admissions committees and mitigates the effect of "moral licensing," or the "subconscious justification of an unfair decision by a failure to recognize what are biased and self-indulgent choices," by admissions committees. (Owen)
- Critical factors for addressing the shortage of Black men in medicine include intervention through pipeline programs, harnessing partnerships and collaborations, leveraging financial resources to expand and maximize opportunities, and building cohorts and using messengers or champions. In particular, Black alumni are an underused resource, which could be empowered and engaged in the efforts to increase the representation of Black men in medicine. (White-Faines)
- Addressing the shortage of Black men in medicine is a matter of will and not knowledge of how or what needs to be done. (White-Faines)
- Through standards, accreditation bodies can guide schools to develop policies, programs, and practices to promote diverse and inclusive academic learning environments. (Catanese)
- It may be necessary to change the predominant narrative equating diversity to underperforming students to students who are high performing and poised to be leaders. (Wilson)

The second day of the meeting began with opening remarks by Cato T. Laurencin, M.D., Ph.D.,[1] and Benjamin S. Carson, Sr., M.D.[2] Laurencin opened the meeting by providing a brief recap of the previous day's discussions and reasserted his call to action to generate ideas and stimulate action to address the shortage of Black men in medicine. Carson provided

[1] Laurencin is university professor, Van Dusen Distinguished Professor of Orthopaedic Surgery, and director, The Raymond and Beverly Sackler Center at the University of Connecticut.

[2] Carson is secretary of the U.S. Department of Housing and Urban Development.

opening comments reflecting on his experience as a medical student and physician, as well as in his current role.

OPENING REMARKS

Benjamin S. Carson, Sr., M.D.
Secretary of Housing and Urban Development

Carson began his remarks by reflecting on his own experience in medical school, the academic challenges he faced, the poor advising, and, ultimately, the realization of how he could best succeed. He spoke of his struggle to learn from lectures and later understanding that he learned better by reading. From that experience, Carson took away the importance of mentoring and tailoring learning to students' needs, including different learning styles. He said,

> When you try to fit yourself into someone else's shoeprint, and you don't really work very well there, you are not going to do well. The sooner we recognize that for everybody, the better off we are going to be. . . . It is up to us to develop it in the right way and to recognize that each individual learns in a different way, and to put the right kind of support there to help people along.

Carson next spoke about his experiences as a pediatric neurosurgeon and struggling with being able to influence only his patients' medical outcomes, especially when they faced challenging life circumstances such as difficult home and family environments outside of the hospital. He expanded on the importance of addressing social determinants and opportunities to intervene on these determinants, such as through housing initiatives. Carson then described initiatives he oversees at the U.S. Department of Housing and Urban Development that can help to improve these social circumstances. He discussed how EnVision Centers, for example, can expose children living in low-income neighborhoods to positive examples of the professions they can aspire to, the many potential pathways to achieving career goals, facilitate mentoring, and provide educational opportunities, including exposure to science, technology, engineering, and mathematics (STEM).[3] Describing the goals of these centers, he asserted,

> It is really about finding ways to get people out of poverty . . . then when they start climbing that ladder of opportunity, not to yank the support

[3] For more information on the EnVision Centers, see https://www.hud.gov/envisioncenters (accessed March 7, 2018).

> so quickly. . . . You have to let them climb high up on that ladder and let that be an advantage that other people will see.

Carson finished his remarks by emphasizing the need to tap into the potential of Black boys and men, which is lost as they leak out of the educational pipeline. He suggested that this lost potential makes the U.S. workforce less competitive globally, and declared,

> We have a responsibility to study history, to understand it, to understand compassion, and to understand that we only have 330 million people in this country, and we have to compete with countries that have four times that many people. We need to develop all of our people, if we are going to be successful in the future.

ACCOUNTABILITY IN MEDICINE

The first panel of the day discussed accountability in medicine, or, what medical schools can do to address the shortage of Black men in medicine. David Acosta, M.D.,[4] launched the panel by putting forward the objective to address what the responsibility is for organizations in addressing the dearth of Black men in medicine, and asked who holds medical schools accountable. He then described different types of accountability, including

- Social accountability, or, the social contract academic health centers have with local and regional communities;
- National accountability for a sufficient and prepared health workforce;
- Compliance accountability for meeting accreditation standards; and
- Internal accountability of each academic health center to its own mission and values.

Finally, Acosta suggested a need to think about the role of other stakeholders not present in the room—for example, local and regional hospitals, hospital associations, pharmaceutical and other industries, and community agencies.

M. Roy Wilson, M.D.,[5] described pipeline programs on his campus. Dimitri T. Azar, M.D., M.B.A.,[6] discussed pipeline programs at the Uni-

[4] Acosta is chief diversity and inclusion officer at the Association of American Medical Colleges.

[5] Wilson is president of Wayne State University.

[6] Azar is executive dean of the University of Illinois College of Medicine and senior director of Patient-Centered Innovation at Google/Verily Life Sciences.

versity of Illinois College of Medicine and the potential for technological solutions. William Owen, M.D., FACP,[7] described how Ross University holds itself accountable for diversity in its student body. Adrienne White-Faines, M.P.A., FACHE,[8] offered reflections on the approach to diversity in osteopathic medicine. Veronica Catanese, M.D., M.B.A.,[9] described how an accrediting body can guide schools to achieve national standards for diversity and pipeline programs. Acosta led a brief discussion following the presentations.

Wayne State University Pipeline Programs

M. Roy Wilson, M.D.
President
Wayne State University

Wilson described initiatives at Wayne State University to address the low college attendance and graduation rates among African Americans. Wayne State University first implemented a student network, a pilot program that offered support for 50 African American male students. The program provided a physical space for the students to gather, study together, and support each other. The network also connected students to Black alumni, faculty, staff, and peer mentors and hosts events like social gatherings, networking opportunities, invited speakers, and field trips. Wilson summed up the effort, saying, "We provide the infrastructure and the structure for them to get together and support each other . . . where they come and they study together. They form a learning community." Wilson reported that the network increased the retention rate between freshman and sophomore years from approximately 60 percent to 95 percent. Based on the success of the program, Wayne State University scaled up the initiative to include all Black male students in the Student African American Brotherhood.[10]

Despite the success of programs like the network and the Brotherhood at Wayne State University, Wilson acknowledged that undergraduate college students are a relatively successful group and that programs at the undergraduate level are late in the pipeline to intervene. Thus, he cautioned that there remains a need to look at the challenges African American boys face before they get to college. To that end, he raised the

[7] Owen is dean and chancellor of the Ross University School of Medicine.

[8] White-Faines is chief executive officer of the American Osteopathic Association.

[9] Catanese is co-secretary of the Liaison Committee on Medical Education (LCME).

[10] For more information on the Wayne State University Student African American Brotherhood, see http://blogs.wayne.edu/saabwsu (accessed March 6, 2018).

conflation of U.S.- and foreign-born Blacks as a challenge, saying, "When we talk about African American, we typically talk about Black." He proceeded to describe the need to distinguish U.S.-born Black students from foreign-born Black students, because the educational achievement and health disparities experienced by native-born Blacks are the result of a legacy of disadvantage and discrimination in the United States. By contrast, foreign-born Blacks have educational and sociocultural experiences that may not be comparable, and which in some instances may reflect privilege. He noted that a similar situation is seen among Hispanic students, where the educational and life experiences of U.S.-born Hispanic students differs from those from Spain and South America. Thus, he encouraged disaggregating data within racial and ethnic groups to parse and better understand the differences in educational achievement between racial and ethnic subgroups.

University of Illinois College of Medicine Pipeline Programs and Potential for New Technology

Dimitri T. Azar, M.D., M.B.A.
Executive Dean, University of Illinois College of Medicine
Senior Director of Patient-Centered Innovation, Google/Verily Life Sciences

Azar began by describing the highly diverse student body at the University of Illinois College of Medicine, of which 25 to 30 percent come from underrepresented minority groups. He attributed this diversity to the school's faculty, a commitment to diversity, a focus on excellence, and the work of the current and past associate deans for diversity and inclusion. Azar also underscored the need to value education:

> We have to work on emphasizing the value of education. I notice when I am talking to those kids who, like me, studied in another country, and their parents came here [from another country], that the value of education is engrained in the mind of the students. Somehow, we are not trying to do [this] to our kids at home, and then we find out that they are interested in other stuff than education. None of them want to go to medical school because it may be tough. But it is important, I think.

Azar then described the strategies the University of Illinois College of Medicine employs to strengthen the medical education pipeline. These include postbaccalaureate programs and summer prematriculation programs prior to entering medical and dental schools as well as managing students' financial issues and wellness programs to address social and economic issues for current medical students. The university also promotes role modeling and mentorship, not only to support students, but by promoting faculty from underrepresented minority backgrounds to become leaders and role models. Finally, for students who do not match into residency programs, the college pays loans and interest for 1 year after graduation. Azar commented that the school has not made any payments to date and that he hopes it will not have to. Instead, the school's primary focus is on preparing students to transition to residencies. Thus, this program serves as a financial incentive, or a mechanism for the school to hold itself financially accountable for better preparing its students.

Reflecting on his experience working simultaneously at the University of Illinois and at Google, Azar noted that the underrepresentation of Black men is common to both settings—academia and technology. Thus, he suggested that efforts to attract, train, and retain underrepresented minorities in both sectors will require systems-based and culturally based solutions, as well as strong role modeling. He commented:

> We have discussed several examples of our effort to solve the problems of attracting, retaining, and training minority medical students. They are not different from the other solutions that, as you have seen, I have mentioned earlier. But they are systems based, if you are thinking about ways to combat, for example, racism, cultural based, trying to change the social systems and so on, and focusing on this individual encouragement and role modeling. But they are all grassroots efforts. For every student, it requires the work of 10 other people perhaps.

Azar discussed the potential for solutions from new technologies to address the shortage of Black men in medicine—for example, how pipeline programs can use data and new technologies, virtual programs, and analytics. He concluded his presentation by challenging those in attendance:

> How can Silicon Valley help to enhance the solutions that have been proposed in this workshop to address the crisis of the growing absence of Black men in medicine and science? How can Silicon Valley attract more Black men to work in data and technology careers, especially health IT [information technology]? And how can they help us improve the pipeline programs and other strategies to address the medical education system, to address cultural norms and values, and to support individual students?

Elements of Accountability for Diversity at the Ross University School of Medicine

William Owen, M.D., FACP
Dean and Chancellor
Ross University School of Medicine

Owen opened his talk by presenting his "organizational credo" for the Ross University School of Medicine: "Attending medical school is not a privilege, but a right for all eligible students." He added that the challenge of this credo is how to define *eligibility*. At Ross, *eligibility* is operationalized as using holistic selection criteria. He expanded, "We manage eligibility for admissions to our own expectations. . . . We also treat applying to medical school as an opportunity to prepare the applicant to become a matriculate." Some of these accepted students are underrepresented minorities with substantially lower Medical College Admission Test (MCAT) scores and grade point averages compared with more traditional and "overwhelmingly Caucasian" applicants. To support them, Ross places these students in a "medical education readiness program" that provides preparatory work during the first few semesters of medical school and also "teaches them how to study." These students are also connected to mentors from a similar background.

Owen identified commitment from leadership as key to increasing diversity at Ross University. He said,

> What is most impactful at Ross for accountability and diversity is that it percolates into the organization from the top, from the board of trustees. [Management consultant] Peter Drucker said eloquently and simplistically, "Trees die from the top." So the mandate for minority success and access at Ross comes from the top, comes from the board of trustees. It comes from the bosses.

Owen described the inclusion of diversity as a key performance indicator for the school. He added that recruitment and retention of underrepresented minorities are monitored over time, and placement rates are benchmarked and discussed at the highest level of the organization, including among trustees. He added that having accountability at the level of leadership removes the responsibility for increasing diversity at the level of admissions committees, saying

> This board of trustees [top]-down approach for accountability mitigates the effect of moral licensing: . . . [the] subconscious justification of an unfair decision by a failure to recognize what are biased and self-indulgent choices occurring by admissions committees.

Owen reflected on his experience being held accountable for diversity. He recalled interviewing as a candidate to become dean when a member of the board of trustees asked, "How do you feel about diversity?" He said,

> A school that is tolerant of moral licensing would be okay if I gave a lukewarm response about diversity. But such tolerance at Ross is a virtual prediction of leadership failure, much like the rejection of a foreign tissue because it is in our DNA. Ross trustees would not accept an organizational leader who is anything less than a zealot for inclusion. So in hindsight, I think I gave the right answer to the trustee's surprising question when I said to him, "Oh, I love diversity." I see it every day when I look in the mirror.

Reflections on Diversity in Osteopathic Medical Schools

Adrienne White-Faines, M.P.A., FACHE
Chief Executive Officer
American Osteopathic Association

White-Faines started her talk by proposing that U.S. osteopathic medical schools, with their more holistic philosophy on patient care and abolitionist roots, are well positioned to promote and improve upon diversity within the U.S. physician workforce. She reminded the audience that the growth and evolution of osteopathic medical schools now positions D.O. physicians equitably alongside their allopathic counterparts. White-Faines then encouraged the audience that progress occurs when there is "the will" to change. She offered from personal experience:

> In the 1970s, there was such a movement to oppose women being in colleges. But Amherst, like many liberal arts schools, made an intentional decision that they want women in their colleges. It is time for our schools to make intentional decisions. It is not something to think about. You just do it. And so it is about being honest. It is about being authentic. It is about all of us calling it out when we see it. It is about being intentional. And it is not so much of how or what do we need to do. The question is, "Do we have the will to do it?"

White-Faines finished by identifying her perspective on critical factors to address the shortage of Black men in medicine. They include intervention through pipeline programs, harnessing partnerships and collaborations, and leveraging financial resources to expand and maximize opportunities. She especially emphasized the importance of building cohorts and using messengers or champions. In particular, she offered African

American medical school alumni as an underused resource, which should be empowered and engaged in the efforts to increase the representation of Black men in medicine.

Diversity in the Learning Environment: Liaison Committee on Medical Education Guidance Principles

Veronica Catanese, M.D., M.B.A.
Co-Secretary
Liaison Committee on Medical Education

LCME, co-sponsored by the American Association of Medical Colleges and the American Medical Association, is the accrediting body for medical education programs leading to a medical doctorate, M.D., degree in the United States and Canada. Of note, accreditation directly targets medical education programs (and indirectly the physicians they produce), whereas certification targets individuals. The LCME accreditation process involves self-study and peer review to determine whether a medical school meets nationally accepted standards of medical education program quality. LCME standards are "concise statements of the expected level of quality or attainment" and comprise elements, or "components that collectively constitute a standard; operationally, elements identify the variables that must be examined to determine a medical education program's compliance with a particular standard." The LCME evaluates each element as "satisfactory," "satisfactory with a need for monitoring," or "unsatisfactory" to inform whether it determines a medical school to be in "compliance," "compliance with monitoring," or "noncompliant" with the each standard.

With regard to the LCME approach to diversity, Catanese focused on the LCME's Standard 3 on academic and learning environments and, specifically, on Element 3.3 on diversity and pipeline programs and partnerships. See Box 7-1 for the LCME Standard 3 and Element 3.3 and Box 7-2 for the criteria by which survey teams assess whether Element 3.3 is satisfactory or not.[11] In summary, Catanese described key elements for schools that meet LCME Standard 3 and Element 3.3, including having mission-appropriate policies and practices to recruit and retain diverse students, faculty, and staff; pipelines and partnerships directed to and focused on identified diversity groups; and evaluation and monitoring processes to assess the effectiveness and progress of those activities. She added that, although her presentation focused on the standard and element directly

[11] For more information on LCME standards and elements, see also http://lcme.org/publications (accessed March 8, 2018).

BOX 7-1
Liaison Committee on Medical Education Standard 3 on Academic and Learning Environments and Element 3.3 on Diversity/Pipeline Programs and Partnerships

Standard 3: Academic and Learning Environments

A medical school ensures that its medical education program occurs in professional, respectful, and intellectually stimulating academic and clinical environments, recognizes the benefits of diversity, and promotes students' attainment of competencies required of future physicians.

3.3 Diversity/Pipeline Programs and Partnerships

A medical school has effective policies and practices in place, and engages in ongoing, systematic, and focused recruitment and retention activities, to achieve mission-appropriate diversity outcomes among its students, faculty, senior administrative staff, and other relevant members of its academic community. These activities include the use of programs and/or partnerships aimed at achieving diversity among qualified applicants for medical school admission and the evaluation of program and partnership outcomes.

SOURCE: Presentation by Veronica Catanese, November 21, 2017.

pertaining to diversity and pipeline programs, diversity also plays a role in other elements of LCME's accreditation—for example, the elements pertaining to professionalism and curricula on cultural competence and health care disparities. She described the intent of LCME to identify the following:

> Diversity practices, policies, and processes [embedded] in an environment that allows them not only to have the desired [diversity] outcomes, but to really have a positive effect on the academic and learning environment of the institution as a whole.

To conclude, Catanese emphasized that LCME seeks to give guidance through its standards and elements, and not to be prescriptive. She said, LCME expects "an institution to really identify its mission-appropriate diversity goals and to direct its resources and attention to achieving them specifically."

BOX 7-2
Liaison Committee on Medical Education Consensus Statement Related to Satisfaction with Element 3.3, Diversity/Pipeline Programs and Partnerships

A. Statement of Satisfactory

Medical education programs will be found to be satisfactory with Element 3.3 when they have all of the following:

- A mission-appropriate diversity policy with identification of diversity groups for students, faculty, and senior administrative staff.
- Ongoing systematic recruitment and retention activities (e.g., pipeline programs and partnerships) to achieve mission-appropriate diversity outcomes in its students, faculty, and senior administrative staff.
- Methods to evaluate the effectiveness of activities to achieve the mission-appropriate diversity outcomes.
- Evidence of effectiveness of the diversity efforts, including offers made and numbers reflecting progress in achieving mission-appropriate diversity outcomes. Evaluation of the sufficiency of the numbers may consider the context of the institution, reasonable timelines for achieving measurable mission-appropriate diversity outcomes, and other supporting data indicative of success in achieving mission-appropriate diversity outcomes.

B. Statement of Satisfactory with a Need for Monitoring

Medical education programs will be found to be satisfactory with a need for monitoring with Element 3.3 when they have satisfactory findings for most areas listed in section A above, but may have one or more of the following:

DISCUSSION

Victoria Mallett, M.D., M.M.M.,[12] inquired about the feasibility of achieving the LCME standards when Blacks are underrepresented at every level of academia. Relatedly, Valerie Montgomery Rice, M.D.,[13] asked whether schools are currently meeting those standards. In response, Wilson described his experience with LCME criteria at Wayne State University School of Medicine. He noted that the M.D. program did not meet LCME criteria in 2014 and it required changing the entire leadership of the medical school to meet the LCME accreditation standard in 2017. He

[12] Mallett is dean of the School of Medicine at Meharry Medical College.

[13] Montgomery Rice is president and dean of the Morehouse School of Medicine.

- Appropriate policies and/or activities so recent as to not yet have demonstrable results.
- Evidence of yearly progress in recruiting and retaining identified diversity groups for students, faculty, and senior administrative staff, but insufficient evidence to demonstrate longer term effectiveness/sustainability of efforts/practices.

C. Statement of Unsatisfactory

Medical education programs will be found to be unsatisfactory with Element 3.3 when they lack one or more of the following:

- A mission-appropriate diversity policy with identification of diversity groups for students, faculty, and senior administrative staff.
- Ongoing systematic recruitment and retention activities (e.g., pipeline programs and partnerships) to achieve mission-appropriate diversity outcomes in its students, faculty, and senior administrative staff.
- Methods to evaluate the effectiveness of activities to achieve the mission-appropriate diversity outcomes.
- Evidence of effective recruitment and retention programs including the offering and acceptance of positions to qualified student, faculty, and staff applicants who are in the school's diversity groups.
- Sufficient progress toward attaining the school's mission-appropriate diversity outcomes.

SOURCES: Presentation by Veronica Catanese, November 21, 2017 and http://lcme.org/publications (accessed March 8, 2018).

added that, within 2 years, Wayne State University School of Medicine went from having 7 underrepresented minorities in the incoming class to having 61. Acosta suggested that medical schools should think about how they can leverage LCME Element 3.3 to enhance their diversity. He pointed out that, according to the standard, schools are asked to define diversity for their institution and identify which population group they will be targeting. Acosta suggested that this would be challenging for those medical schools located in states where the White population is predominant. He challenged these institutions, arguing,

> Many of our schools are land grant public institutions, which means they are not only obligated to their social contract with their local and regional communities and state, but also to the nation itself.

Acosta acknowledged that LCME can only offer guidance, and how it guides medical schools is important. He noted that when LCME cited the medical school he was working at as "satisfactory with a need for monitoring" on Element 3.3, this gave him the leverage to make diversity a priority among leadership. Catanese commented about the importance of thinking broadly about pipelines and the total academic environment, which includes not only students, but also faculty, once these students enter an academic career. Acosta added that this academic environment includes not only students and faculty, but also staff. Finally, White-Faines proposed the need to think longitudinally over time and echoed Acosta's call to think of failing to achieve LCME elements not as a fault, but an opportunity. She said,

> Yesterday's standards may not apply today. So I think everyone should walk away feeling like they have a right, even though [LCME] says everybody can appeal to the standards review, but really use that leverage to say, here is an opportunity for us. Together, we can work on both sides of the process to bring in and think about what does the faculty of tomorrow look like, and how do we need to redefine it as opposed to you won't let me. Let's make it work for us.

George Hill, Ph.D.,[14] endorsed funding and dedicating resources to increasing mentoring networks and developing new ideas for mentoring. He also inquired about whether mentors in programs discussed were necessarily Black. Azar said, regarding the importance of the quality of mentors, "There were many mentors who just thought it was a good idea to be a mentor. And so they are lousy mentors. And just because their skin color matches the color of the person they are mentoring is not sufficient." To address this challenge, he developed a program called "Mentor the Mentor" to guide interested mentors in how best to do so and to ensure that well-intentioned mentors do not inadvertently harm their mentees.

Laurencin reflected on what he took away from the panel. First, he described the need to replicate successful pipeline programs, such as the one Wilson described at Wayne State University. Second, he elaborated on White-Faines's comment about the need to make intentional decisions to address the dearth of Black men in medicine. Drawing a parallel to the increased awareness about sexual harassment and the #metoo movement, he remarked,

[14] Hill is Levi Watkins Jr., M.D. professor emeritus in medical education, distinguished professor of pathology, medicine, and immunology emeritus, and past vice chancellor for equity, diversity, and inclusion, and chief diversity officer at Vanderbilt University.

> The fact is, 20 years ago, sexual harassment was around. But it wasn't on the front page of *The New York Times* like it is today. And so one of the things that happened was there was a cacophony of discussion that started happening around this. People said this is not acceptable. We are going to call it what it is, and changes are going to occur. We have to have that same concept of having that same cacophony of thought and discussion to bring this to the fore to make a big difference.

Third, he reacted to Azar's comments on the potential of new technologies and emphasized the need to harness technology and to use it to identify potential students.

In closing, Owen asked Wilson whether there is a need to groom leaders. Wilson responded by describing a program that changes the narrative equating diversity to underperforming students to students who are exceptionally well prepared and already poised to be leaders. He described responding negatively to a proposal that addressed lack of diversity with postbaccalaureate programs, and feeling bothered by the traditional narrative of students in postbaccalaureate programs as being behind or deficient in some way, and having the stigma of needing extra help. In response, he created a program called Med-Direct,[15] which offers admission to the undergraduate school and the medical school at Wayne State University for high-performing high school students. The program covers tuition and housing for undergraduate students and tuition for medical students for a cohort of 10 students annually and is intended to lead to an M.D. or a M.D./Ph.D. degree program also at Wayne State University. The program also provides opportunities for research, MCAT and Graduate Record Examinations preparation, and summer enrichment courses including leadership development, as well as seminars, workshops, and clinical training in the School of Medicine during the academic year. In closing, he reiterated the idea that this program challenges the perception that pipeline programs for students from diverse backgrounds are postbaccalaureate programs for students struggling to get into medical schools. Instead, it offers the narrative that they are for high performing students who are well positioned to become future physician leaders.

[15] For more information on Wayne Med-Direct, see https://provost.wayne.edu/workforce-diversity/wayne-med-direct (accessed March 9, 2018).

8

Financial Barriers to Medical Education

Highlights Presented by Individual Speakers

- Financial barriers to medical education include not only medical school tuition, but also costs related to applying to schools, preparing for and taking standardized tests, and tuition for schooling prior to medical school. Not only do individual students bear these costs, but their families do, as well. (Knight)
- Financing medical education can be a psychological barrier in addition to a material one. (Dyer, Knight)
- Financial crises not involving education-related costs (e.g., medical expenses, temporary homelessness, and childcare emergencies) can threaten students' continuation in medical school. (Dyer)
- Financial barriers occur in the context of other challenges like systemic racism, a lack of opportunity or role models, and negative social norms and values of Black men. (Knight)
- Teaching financial literacy may help students make better financial decisions. Incorporating financial literacy in mentoring should begin at earlier ages, such as among high school seniors taking on undergraduate loans. (Mallett)
- Financial costs may be especially burdensome for those who discontinue their medical education. (Knight)

This panel focused on the financial barriers Black boys and men face throughout the medical education trajectory, and discussed potential opportunities to address these barriers. Esther R. Dyer, M.L.S., D.L.S.,[1] described scholarships and other funding that the National Medical Fellowships (NMF) provide to underrepresented minorities in health professional education. Joseph B. Hill[2] discussed a unique collaboration between the Thomas Jefferson University and Alpha Boulé chapter of the Sigma Pi Phi fraternity, to support a medical education pipeline program. Michael Knight, M.D.,[3] offered insight from his experience into the perceived financial barriers from the student perspective. Theodore Corbin, M.D., M.P.P.,[4] led a brief discussion following the presentations.

NATIONAL MEDICAL FELLOWSHIPS

Esther R. Dyer, M.L.S., D.L.S.
President and Chief Executive Officer
National Medical Fellowships

NMF is a nonprofit organization that provides scholarships and awards to underrepresented minority medical students and offers service-learning programs to students in the health professions. Franklin McLean, M.D., Ph.D., a physician/researcher who helped found the University of Chicago School of Medicine, established the Fellowships in 1946 in recognition of the lack of opportunities for Black physicians (including no residency programs for Black students at the time) and of the need for Black physicians to ensure access to high-quality health care for all Americans. Originally providing scholarships to only Blacks, NMF opened its funding to other underrepresented groups in the health professions in 1968. The organization aims "to identify and nurture talent early, to provide opportunities to level the playing field, and to be a good investment in the future of health care," Dyer said.

Dyer provided a brief overview of the financial burdens of medical education, including application, tuition, and examination costs, as well as the resulting debt. She also described financing medical education as a

---

[1] Dyer is president and chief executive officer of the National Medical Fellowships.

[2] Hill is senior vice president and diversity officer, Enterprise Office of Diversity, Inclusion, and Community Engagement at Thomas Jefferson University and Jefferson Health and Alpha Boulé chapter of the Sigma Pi Phi fraternity.

[3] Knight is assistant professor of medicine and patient safety officer, Division of General Internal Medicine at The George Washington University and former president of the Student National Medical Association.

[4] Corbin is vice chair for research and associate professor in the Department of Emergency Medicine at the Drexel University College of Medicine.

psychological barrier among underrepresented minorities and how NMF can help students overcome this challenge, saying,

> They need guidance and support to understand how they can achieve their dreams and their passions, and walking the paths that you [as African American leaders in medicine] have walked, and still manage to feed their families and eventually retire.

Dyer briefly discussed two of NMF's programs, the Dr. David Monash/Harry Lloyd and Elizabeth Pawlette Marshall Medical Student Scholarship Program and the Primary Care Leadership Program. The former provides service scholarships to 1st-year through 3rd-year medical students to conduct a community health project and residency scholarships of $25,000 to decrease medical school debt to 4th-year medical students who are matched as clinical residents in the Chicago area and who exhibit a commitment to serving underserved populations in Chicago.[5] The Primary Care Leadership Program places 2nd-year and 3rd-year medical students, graduate nursing students, and graduate physician assistant students in partnering community health centers (CHCs). The program offers scholarship funding, mentoring, exposure to primary care, and the opportunity to make an impact in these CHCs.[6]

NMF also has an Emergency Scholarship Program, which provides bridge funding for students for whom financial crises threaten their continuation in medical school.[7] These often-unexpected crises typically involve non-education-related costs—for example, medical expenses, temporary homelessness, childcare emergencies, and other crises. These funds also support 4th-year medical students' costs related to securing a residency (e.g., application fees, travel to interviews). Dyer offered examples of emergency scholarship recipients. Lagu Androga, a 3rd-year medical student at Albert Einstein College of Medicine, had an untreated eye problem that hindered his ability to pass his medical licensing step examinations. The NMF Emergency Scholarship Program supported a preparation course for Androga to pass the exams. Trevor York, a 4th-year student at the University of Buffalo State University of New York School

[5] For more information on the Dr. David Monash/Harry Lloyd and Elizabeth Pawlette Marshall Medical Student Scholarship Program, see https://nmfonline.org/about-our-scholarships-and-awards/service-learning-programs/monashscott-medical-student-scholarship-program (accessed March 9, 2018).

[6] For more information on the NMF Primary Care Leadership Program, see https://nmfonline.org/about-our-scholarships-and-awards/service-learning-programs/nmf-primary-care-leadership-program (accessed March 9, 2018).

[7] For more information on the NMF Emergency Scholarship Fund, see https://nmfonline.org/about-our-scholarships-and-awards/nmf-emergency-scholarship-fund (accessed March 9, 2018).

of Medicine and Biomedical Sciences, was raised by a sick, single mother with no medical coverage or funds to pay for medical care. This experience inspired him to become a physician, but, by his 3rd year of medical school, he had only $500 in savings and increasing debt. Additionally, after setbacks in his medical school rotations, York needed to take time off to receive counseling. When York returned to his studies, he rebounded academically, but lacked funds to pay for basic costs—food, electricity, and rent. The NMF Fellowship offered him bridge funding for these costs and also to support travel to take his medical licensing step examination and to travel to interview for residency programs. Currently, he is a recipient of the NMF National Alumni Council scholarship and is in the process of identifying his residency options.

To close, Dyer presented a quote from Marcus Rushing, a 2012 recipient of the United Health Foundation/NMF Diverse Medical Scholars Program and a member of the NMF Young Alumni Leadership Council: "NMF provided me with financial support, and they gave me one of the greatest gifts that you can ever give a person: they gave me an opportunity." Dyer reiterated that, in addition to funding, NMF offers support and opportunity. She said, "We [NMF] believe in them, and that this is an opportunity for them to be successful, and that we recognize that."

THE JACKSON/MINTON SCHOLARSHIP FUND

Joseph B. Hill
Senior Vice President and Chief Diversity Officer
Enterprise Office of Diversity, Inclusion, and Community Engagement
Thomas Jefferson University and Jefferson Health System

The Jackson/Minton Scholarship Fund provides scholarship funding to Black men to promote diversity at Thomas Jefferson University Sidney Kimmel Medical College.[8] Hill recalled the dean of the college directing him to increase recruitment of Black men to the school upon his arrival at Jefferson. Looking into the history of the university, Hill discovered that the first Black graduate from Jefferson Medical College was Algernon Brashear Jackson in 1901. Together, Jackson and fellow African American Jefferson Medical College alumnus Henry McKee Minton founded Sigma Pi Phi, also known as the Boulé, a fraternal organization composed of prominent Black men, many of whom have been or are leaders in advocating for civil rights, social justice, economic and educational equality, and which offers professional and social support for Black professionals,

[8] For more information, see https://w3.jefferson.edu/giving/sigma-pi-phi.html (accessed March 9, 2018).

including mentoring and fellowships for young Black men.[9] This history spurred Hill to reach out to the Sigma Pi Phi to create a Jackson/Minton Scholarship for African American men at the Sidney Kimmel Medical College. With additional matched funding from the Sidney Kimmel Foundation, which generously supports the Jefferson Medical College more broadly, the Sidney Kimmel Medical College together with Sigma Pi Phi launched the Jackson/Minton Scholarship during the Democratic National Convention in Philadelphia in 2016.

While conducting initial fundraising in collaboration with the Boulé Foundation, several Boulé members who were also Jefferson Medical College alumni recalled the challenges and barriers they faced as students. Spurred by these comments, Hill expanded the fellowship to include a mentoring program featuring members of the Alpha Boulé chapter (of Philadelphia), to help guide students through the medical school experience. The goals of the Jackson/Minton Scholarship are to

- Create a $1 million endowed scholarship (matched by the Sidney Kimmel Foundation for a total endowment of $2 million);
- Increase enrollment of Black men at the Sidney Kimmel Medical College; and
- Provide mentors from among members of the Sigma Pi Phi Boulé to scholarship recipients.

The scholarship also aims to support the Summer Training and Enrichment Program for Underrepresented Persons (STEP-UP) Medicine pipeline program at Sidney Kimmel Medical College. The STEP-UP program is a comprehensive summer enrichment program for undergraduate students from groups underrepresented in the medical professions and from economically disadvantaged backgrounds who intend to apply to medical school.[10] It provides preparation for the Medical College Admission Test (MCAT) and for the medical school application process; enrichment programs on health policy, health disparities, and health equity; and experiences in clinical shadowing and workshops on medical skills.

Hill finished his presentation by remarking,

> We wanted to make a difference. Here is an opportunity for successful African American males, most [of whom] are already physicians, to really give back and to really start identifying more African American males [to] come to Thomas Jefferson [University].

---

[9] For more information about Sigma Pi Phi, see https://www.sigmapiphi.org/home (accessed May 3, 2018).

[10] For more information on the STEP-UP program, see http://www.jefferson.edu/university/diversity/pipeline_programs/step_up.html (accessed March 9, 2018).

FINANCIAL BARRIERS TO MEDICAL EDUCATION FROM THE STUDENT PERSPECTIVE

Michael Knight, M.D.
Assistant Professor of Medicine and Patient Safety Officer
Division of General Internal Medicine
The George Washington University

Knight recalled his experiences and the experiences of fellow Black medical students he represented from his former tenure as president of the Student National Medical Association. He urged the audience to think about financial barriers early in the pipeline, starting with the costs of preparing for and taking the SAT in high school, college applications, undergraduate tuition and loans, applying to medical school (including preparing for and taking the MCATs and travel for interviews), medical school tuition, and through the costs of applying to residency programs. He described these as costs not only for individual students, but also for their families who may be financially supporting students through their schooling. He remarked,

> We have to think about the challenges that families are going through. My own family [took on] thousands of dollars in credit card debt just [for me] to take the MCAT, just to go on interviews. Thank God I made it and got to medical school and actually have been able to give back, so we could pay that off.

He expanded on the financial burdens on those who discontinue medical education and how seeing the costs for these students who discontinue their education can discourage others. He commented,

> There are many of us that don't make it. And when you see other students who have tried to go to medical school, and they are not successful, and they are still stuck with that debt, what incentive is it for me to go down that same path?

Knight also encouraged the audience to think about financial barriers in the context of other challenges. He described lack of opportunity, systemic racism, low expectations, and negative portrayals of Black boys and men in the media. He described the lack of role models as an incentive to pursue medical careers. Recalling his own experience, he said,

> No one in the family is a physician. No one at church is a physician. Sometimes these opportunities are not even realities. When we go to school and are told, "Boys do this," the incentive to excel in your

> academics—in science, in mathematics—is not there. If you are not seeing these examples, what is the incentive for us to pursue these careers?

For those who graduate college and are accepted to medical school, Knight described the cost of graduate medical education as a psychological barrier. He said,

> When you are coming from a family that is hardly making anything, thinking about a loan in the hundreds of thousands, yes, you are going to be a physician. You are going to be able to pay it back. But think of coming from a family where no one has even had $100,000 in any bank account or anything such as that. You are signing up for a loan for $300,000. Just think of what that is doing to your mind and what that is doing to your incentive to even pursue this.

Knight concluded his presentation by describing the need to increase access to existing scholarships. Although many scholarships exist, knowledge of them does not necessarily reach many young students who are interested in pursuing health careers. He underscored the need to help young Black boys to navigate the medical education process and to alert them to available opportunities—financial and otherwise—to ensure this interest and potential is not lost. He closed his presentation by posing the question,

> [Who] we are not seeing make it are those who are at the most risk that don't have those support systems. How can we utilize our resources to really affect and change the lives of those who are most in need?

DISCUSSION

Cato T. Laurencin, M.D., Ph.D.,[11] raised the issue of what to do for students who discontinue their medical education, either who leave schooling before graduating or who complete medical school but do not match with a residency program. He also urged further consideration of costs unrelated to education, but instead related to family and social issues that can be financial burdens and barriers, the "mental anguish" these financial situations create, and their consequences for academic performance. Hill responded, "When [students] start medical school, the family issues, the social issues, don't stop. Many times, they get worse." He added that people often justify the high costs of medical education with the high

[11] Laurencin is university professor, Van Dusen Distinguished Professor of Orthopaedic Surgery, and director, The Raymond and Beverly Sackler Center at the University of Connecticut.

salaries of physicians. However, this premise may not be realistic for individuals whose life circumstances make it difficult to complete their medical education and become physicians on the expected timeline.

William Owen, M.D., FACP,[12] raised the potential of financial literacy programs. He commented that even for students who receive educational loans, often they do not know how to handle money and consequently increase their debt. Building on this comment, Victoria Mallett, M.D., M.M.M.,[13] raised the need for financial literacy at an even younger age. Underrepresented minority students often come to medical school with greater indebtedness from their undergraduate education. She therefore suggested the need to look at incorporating financial literacy in mentoring and to examine financial decision making among high school seniors taking on undergraduate loans. Recalling her experience with boys her family took in, she said

> It was amazing to me when my "bonus sons" were in undergrad and getting their loans, they would talk about their refunds. I said, "That is not a refund. That is a loan that you have to pay back. And you will be saddled with it your whole life, because there is no bankruptcy. There is no forgiveness. You can never get out of this." . . . Try to get a 17-year old to understand this. Since when do 17-year olds get to make a $100,000 decision? The banks have set this up, and we have allowed them to do that.

[12] Owen is dean and chancellor of the Ross University School of Medicine.

[13] Mallett is dean of the School of Medicine at Meharry Medical College.

9

Approaches from Philanthropy

Highlights Presented by Individual Speakers

- The Burroughs Wellcome Fund employs the key strategies of exposure, enrichment, engagement, and enrollment to promote leadership and empowerment among youth. (Mays)
- A philosophy of engaging students' minds and incorporating academic and professional development as tools to aid students in becoming successful leaders is critical to the Burroughs Wellcome Fund approach to awarding grants along the medical educational and career trajectory. (Mays)
- For The Commonwealth Fund, investing in human capital is a key strategy to achieve its goal to improve the health system for vulnerable populations. (Blumenthal)
- Opportunities to increase diversity beyond focusing on increasing the number of Black men in medical schools at different junctures along the medical educational trajectory are important to consider. (Blumenthal)
- Several ideas to challenge traditional thinking about pipeline programs include increasing partnerships with community colleges, more research on the role of diversity in improving the medical education experience of all students, and developing a language that engages a broader section of the population and builds relationships rather than divisiveness. (Lumpkin)

The philanthropy panel discussed grant making as a tool to strengthen the medical education pipeline and to promote diversity in the health workforce. Alfred M. Mays, M.S.,[1] discussed programs under the Science Education and Diversity in Science portfolios at the Fund. David Blumenthal, M.D., M.P.P.,[2] described pipeline programs and programs to improve the health of vulnerable populations that The Commonwealth Fund currently supports and has supported historically. John Lumpkin, M.D., M.P.H.,[3] discussed the pipeline programs supported by RWJF and offered ideas to challenge the traditional thinking about these programs.[4] Cedric M. Bright, M.D., FACP,[5] led a brief discussion following the presentations.

BURROUGHS WELLCOME FUND

Alfred M. Mays, M.S.
Program Officer, Science Education and Diversity in Science
Burroughs Wellcome Fund

BWF is an independent private foundation that supports science research and education to advance the biomedical sciences. As the program officer responsible for the Fund's portfolios on science education and diversity in science, Mays oversees approximately 14 percent of the Fund's grant making. The mission of the Diversity in Science portfolio is "to increase the number of underrepresented minority scientists within the biomedical and medical research and education community through career enrichment and mentoring support," he said. The Fund supports several initiatives to achieve this goal. The Postdoctoral Enrichment Program awards $60,000 of supplemental funding for underrepresented minority postdoctoral fellows.[6] This funding does not support the awardee's research position, but rather seeks to support career development through engagement and affiliation with major associations and mentor workshops, including online modules and webinars.

---

[1] Mays is program officer at the Burroughs Wellcome Fund (BWF).

[2] Blumenthal is president of The Commonwealth Fund.

[3] Lumpkin is senior vice president at the Robert Wood Johnson Foundation (RWJF).

[4] For information on BWF, see https://www.bwfund.org (accessed April 30, 2018), The Commonwealth Fund, see http://www.commonwealthfund.org (accessed April 30, 2018), and RWJF, see https://www.rwjf.org (accessed April 30, 2018).

[5] Bright is associate dean for inclusive excellence, director of the Office of Special Programs, and associate professor of medicine at the University of North Carolina School of Medicine.

[6] For more information on the BWF Postdoctoral Enrichment Program, see https://www.bwfund.org/grant-programs/diversity-science/postdoctoral-enrichment-program (accessed March 12, 2018).

The Graduate Diversity Enrichment Program awards $5,000 over 2 years to support underrepresented minority Ph.D. candidates enrolled in a North Carolina university and who are conducting biomedical research.[7] This pilot program seeks to provide similar support as the postdoctoral program, but for students in the graduate level. Key to these programs are effective mentorships. To foster such mentorships, BWF engages the Center for the Improvement of Mentored Experiences in Research to conduct cultural diversity training and mentorship workshops for the BWF Postdoctoral Enrichment Program Fellows in collaboration with the Howard Hughes Medical Institute Gilliam Fellows.[8] BWF also funds a range of ad hoc programs to increase diversity in science, including efforts to replicate the Meyerhoff Scholars Program at the University of Maryland, Baltimore County,[9] and a Diversity in Science, Technology, Engineering, and Mathematics (STEM) speaker series.

The mission of the BWF Science Education program is "to build systematic reform in science, technology, engineering, and mathematics primarily in North Carolina," Mays said. This portfolio includes a range of activities covering informal and formal education programs, public policy and research efforts, and capacity and partnership building programs. Mays highlighted several programs, including a STEM Funders Network, a group of approximately 30 funders collaborating to support a national STEM ecosystem, and the North Carolina Science, Mathematics, and Technology (SMT) Center, a nonprofit organization that promotes quality STEM education in North Carolina.

In one initiative, the SMT Center along with other stakeholders identified key attributes of a STEM education, which the North Carolina State Board of Education adopted as the standard measure of quality STEM education programs in the state. This stakeholder group also developed STEM Implementation Rubrics to guide schools to implement quality STEM programs. As a further resource, the SMT Center hosts the North Carolina STEM Learning Network, a partnership with the North Carolina Department of Public Instruction, the Community College System, independent colleges and universities in the state, and others, where educators throughout the state can find and share programs and opportunities related to STEM education.[10]

---

[7] For more information on the BWF Graduate Diversity Enrichment Program, see https://www.bwfund.org/grant-programs/diversity-science/graduate-diversity-enrichment-program (accessed March 12, 2019).

[8] For more information on the Center for the Improvement of Mentored Experiences in Research, see https://cimerproject.org/# (accessed March 12, 2018).

[9] See Chapter 5 for more discussion of the Meyerhoff Scholars Program.

[10] For more information on the North Carolina STEM Learning Network, see https://www.ncsmt.org/programs/nc-stem-learning-network (accessed March 12, 2018).

In closing, Mays described the Fund's "4-E Strategy" to promote leadership and empowerment among youth, which comprises exposure, enrichment, engagement, and enrollment. He added, "When we build programs, we actually follow that model to expose, to enrich, to engage, and then our metric is the enrollment." Finally, he underscored BWF's approach to award grants along the medical educational and career trajectory, its philosophy of "strategies that engage minds," and the importance of incorporating academic and professional development as tools to aid students in becoming successful leaders.

THE COMMONWEALTH FUND

David Blumenthal, M.D., M.P.P.
President
The Commonwealth Fund

The Commonwealth Fund is a private foundation that seeks to promote a high-performing health system. Its portfolio focuses on improving the health system for vulnerable populations, which the Fund achieves through two streams of grant making—investing in human capital and delivery system reform. Discussing grant making in the human capital investments stream, Blumenthal first presented three Fund-supported programs to advance the careers of Black men in science and medicine. Since 1949, the Fund has provided grant support to the National Medical Fellowships (NMF). As Esther Dyer, M.L.S., D.L.S.,[11] described in the panel on financial barriers to medical education, NMF provides a range of scholarships for underrepresented minorities as they pursue their medical education.[12]

In 1968, the Fund awarded Meharry Medical College a $700,000 grant (approximately $5 million in current U.S. dollars) to improve graduate-level education in the basic sciences. Finally, in 1996, the Fund established the Mongan Fellowship in Minority Health Policy. As described in detail in the session on current medical pipeline strategies, Blumenthal emphasized that the Fellowship is especially committed to "recruiting and cultivating physicians who are intent on being leaders in the promotion of minority health and the interest of disadvantaged populations." He elaborated that fellowship alumni have gone on to become not only leaders in academia, but also the public sector, with program graduates becoming directors of state and local health departments.

---

[11] Dyer is president and chief executive officer of NMF.

[12] See Chapter 8 for discussion on the history and current programs of the National Medical Fellowships.

Blumenthal discussed the importance of thinking about different junctures along the medical educational trajectory, and not focusing solely on increasing the number of Black men in medical schools. He said of the Mongan Fellowships, "It is not about getting people into medical school, but it is about taking the graduates of medical schools to another level where they can become role models for people who would follow them along the way." Since its founding, the Fund has awarded more than 120 fellowships.[13]

Blumenthal next briefly presented several Commonwealth Fund initiatives in its delivery system reform stream of grant making. Speaking about the goals of these efforts, he said

> [These delivery system reforms seek] to promote the health of minority populations by making sure that the health system serves their needs directly and appropriately. That . . . is our primary way . . . in which we serve the interests, not only of African American males, but also African American females and Hispanics and other minority populations.

He described the Fund's work on coverage and access, to reduce rates of uninsurance among vulnerable populations, especially with the implementation of the Patient Protection and Affordable Care Act of 2010. Additionally, Blumenthal described supporting work related to Medicaid (and its expansion) and cross-national work that examines "things that we can import to the United States that may be useful for our delivery system."

ROBERT WOOD JOHNSON FOUNDATION

John Lumpkin, M.D., M.P.H.
Senior Vice President
Robert Wood Johnson Foundation

Lumpkin began his presentation by proposing a new way of thinking about the medical education pipeline. He suggested,

> We really ought to be moving from pipeline as a metaphor to a funnel. . . . We really have to think about the funnel in two ways. One, it begins to direct people to health professions. And the second thing is that the funnel is circular. Because when we think about people moving through the pipeline, if people can not only reach back and reach down, they begin to engage those before them.

[13] See Chapter 5 for additional discussion on the Mongan Fellowships.

To that end, Lumpkin described the RWJF approach to programs to enhance the medical educational pipeline. RWJF seeks not only to increase the number of underrepresented minorities who enter the health professions, but also to develop individuals to become role models to help guide decision making. He elaborated that, not only will addressing the crisis of the dearth of Black men in medicine require new thinking, but solving the crisis will also require new thinking. Paraphrasing Donald Berwick, M.D., M.P.P., FRCP,[14] he said, "Every system is perfectly designed to get the results that it gets." He expanded,

> And what our system does is it has a certain group of individuals in our society who start off behind and they stay behind throughout their life. It is no surprise. These are young African American boys; young people who do not get the opportunity because they enter behind and they stay behind. How do we begin to make a difference? Let's think about where in this pipeline funnel we begin to think about interventions.

Lumpkin then described RWJF-funded interventions along the pipeline/funnel. These include interventions to address adverse childhood experiences, mitigate lead exposure, provide trauma-informed care in early childhood, and support universal pre-kindergarten. For high school students, RWJF supports the Forward Promise program focusing on at-risk youth in high school that "empowers boys and young men of color to heal, to grow, and to thrive and to enter college and be ready to be successful as potential candidates to go on to medical school and to go into the sciences."[15] Lumpkin also described a past program, the Health Professions Partnership Initiative, that partnered medical schools with inner-city high schools. He described the lesson learned from this initiative that it required commitment from the top. He explained,

> If there was commitment by leadership of the top of the medical schools, then these partnerships were successful. But when these partnerships were delegated as far down [the organizational chart] as they could [go, then they] were not successful.

Lumpkin also underscored the importance of high school as an intervention target. He reasoned,

---

[14] Berwick is president emeritus and senior fellow at the Institute for Healthcare Improvement and former administrator of the Centers for Medicare & Medicaid Services.

[15] For more information on Forward Promise, see https://www.rwjf.org/en/how-we-work/grants-explorer/featured-programs/forward-promise.html (accessed March 12, 2018).

> When you compare a young person at age 25 who has not completed high school with someone who has completed college, the difference in life expectancy is 9 years. . . . An early intervention in the child's life that helps them be successful and graduate high school and go to college may be the most impactful thing we can do to increase life expectancy in this country.

At the undergraduate level, Lumpkin described the Summer Medical Professions Education Program, which exposes rising sophomores to the health sciences and provides math and science enrichment.[16] At the graduate level, RWJF supports a new program called the Health Policy Research Scholars, which provides financial support, education, and leadership for underrepresented minority doctoral students in nonclinical health fields.[17] Finally, Lumpkin described the Harold Amos Medical Faculty Development Program, which provides research funding and a stipend to historically disadvantaged physicians, dentists, and nurses to encourage and foster their academic and professional development and to increase the number of health professionals from disadvantaged backgrounds who achieve senior rank in academic medicine, dentistry, and nursing.[18]

In closing, Lumpkin offered several ideas to challenge the traditional thinking about pipeline programs. First, he proposed increasing partnerships with community colleges. Second, he discussed the need for more research on the role of diversity in improving the medical education experience of all students. Finally, he proposed a new way of thinking about and framing the issue of the lack of diversity in medical education, and the dearth of Black men in particular. He asserted,

> Racism is an ideology of division. It splits folks up. As we think about how we are fighting racism, we should be careful about the language that we use. I do not believe that the truth shall set us free. I believe power will set us free. We need to look at the partnerships that we can make in order to have the power to affect the change that we need to see happen. . . . I think we have to be careful about terms such as *white privilege* and *white advantage* because I know, while it does exist, [they are not terms that build] unity and power. It helps focus in on the division. . . . We need to think about not only how we address this issue as we understand it, but to begin to use the language that a broader section of the population

---

[16] For more information on the Summer Health Professions Education Program, see http://www.shpep.org (accessed March 12, 2018).

[17] For more information on the Health Policy Research Scholars, see http://healthpolicyresearch-scholars.org (accessed March 12, 2018).

[18] For more information about the Harold Amos Medical Faculty Development Program, see http://www.amfdp.org (accessed March 12, 2018).

> uses, those who need to be supportive, not put off, to help us address the challenge of increasing the number of African American men in math, science, and medicine.

Lumpkin finished his presentation by paraphrasing Hillel the Elder, the famous Jewish religious leader, asking the audience, "If not us, who? If not now, when?"

DISCUSSION

Deborah Prothrow-Stith, M.D.,[19] asked the panel how they address sustainability in their funding. Blumenthal acknowledged a fundamental tension for philanthropies and described this challenge, stating,

> Sustainability is a challenge for philanthropy because we simply cannot devote ourselves to a couple of programs over centuries and decades. . . . There is a basic dilemma that philanthropy has, which is that it would basically stall as a creative force if it continued to support every program that it funded in any given year.

Mays echoed this challenge, and offered a two-stage approach to giving—first, a phase where a philanthropic organization needs to be able to take risks on initial investments, and second, only moving to support sustainability if those early programs are shown to be effective.

[19] Prothrow-Stith is dean of the College of Medicine at Charles R. Drew University.

10

Approaches from Government

Highlights Presented by Individual Speakers

- Student athletes of the National Collegiate Athletic Association may be a pool of potential medical school students and are worth engaging. (Valantine)
- The myth that successful researchers are necessarily good mentors needs to be challenged. Evidence suggests that this is an incorrect assumption. (Valantine)
- Program evaluations are important; a lack of data because program outcomes are not measured does not necessarily indicate programs do not work. (Valantine)
- Developing a diverse workforce is a priority of the Heath Resources and Services Administration's Bureau of Health Workforce to strengthen the health workforce and to improve the health of underserved and vulnerable populations. (Padilla)
- Tracking and monitoring pipeline program participant outcomes and focusing on community-based training and longitudinal training are potential strategies for moving forward. (Padilla)

This panel featured presentations on strategies to increase diversity of the health workforce from two government agencies and lessons learned.

Elizabeth Ofili, M.D.,[1] moderated the panel and opened the discussion by posing a series of questions. She asked,

> What do you see as the most innovative approaches in your organization to address the problem of the absence of Black men in medicine and science? How is the impact of those efforts assessed? Are there important learnings to date? What is standing in the way of these efforts or challenges, and what new strategies are needed?

Hannah A. Valantine, M.D., M.R.C.P.,[2] described pipeline programs and other approaches to increase diversity in the scientific workforce that the National Institutes of Health (NIH) support. She also proposed engaging the National Collegiate Athletic Association (NCAA) and college athletes as an untapped pool of potential students to enhance the medical school matriculation rates of Black men. Luis Padilla, M.D., FAAFP,[3] discussed priorities and programs regarding the health workforce at the Health Resources and Services Administration's (HRSA's) Bureau of Health Workforce (BHW). Following the presentations, Ofili moderated a brief discussion.

NATIONAL INSTITUTES OF HEALTH AND ENGAGING NEW PARTNERS

Hannah A. Valantine, M.D., M.R.C.P.
Chief Officer, Scientific Workforce Diversity, and Senior Investigator
National Heart, Lung, and Blood Institute

Valantine began her presentation by discussing several initiatives at NIH to increase diversity in their workforce. She first discussed the Building Infrastructure Leading to Diversity (BUILD) program, which awarded grants to 10 undergraduate institutions to research and implement innovative approaches to engaging and sustaining interest in students from diverse backgrounds in biomedical research, beginning in 2014.[4] Eligibility criteria for the program were that an institution received less than $7.5 million in NIH research grants in the preceding year and that 25 percent

---

[1] Ofili is professor of medicine, director of the Clinical Research Center, and senior associate dean of clinical and translational research at Morehouse School of Medicine.

[2] Valantine is chief officer, Scientific Workforce Diversity, and senior investigator at the National Heart, Lung, and Blood Institute.

[3] Padilla is associate administrator of the Health Resources and Services Administration's Bureau of Health Workforce.

[4] For more information on the NIH BUILD Initiative, see https://www.nigms.nih.gov/training/dpc/Pages/build.aspx (accessed March 13, 2018).

of students at the institution receive Pell Grants. The 10 awardees collect data on shared metrics, or "hallmarks of success." To evaluate the BUILD universities' innovative approaches to supporting diversity, the programs were implemented as experiments with two comparison groups—an internal control group and external control group from a non-BUILD institution. NIH also created a Center for Coordination and Evaluation to collect and analyze data from these evaluations to identify what works.

In parallel with the BUILD program, NIH also established a National Research Mentoring Network in 2014.[5] The network connects mentors and mentees in person and online and also offers mentor training led by researcher Christine Pfund, Ph.D., a scientist at the University of Wisconsin, which teaches "people how to become better mentors including culture-sensitive mentoring." Valantine explained the need to challenge "the myth that because you are a good and successful researcher, you are automatically a good mentor. The data has been quite clear that this is an incorrect assumption."

Valantine next described some past NIH programs to promote diversity. She first described the longstanding NIH diversity supplement, an administrative grant supplement that allowed NIH grantees the opportunity to include a person from an underrepresented group, frequently at the graduate or postdoctoral level, to work on the grantee's project. An analysis of the program found that 60 percent of people supported by diversity supplements were performing well and still working in science. Valantine noted that this was contrary to common assumptions about the program, and thus offered "a lesson to all of us that just because something is not measured and the data is not there, it does not mean it does not work." Valantine also mentioned the Bridges to the Baccalaureate Program, which supports linkages between 2-year junior or community colleges and 4-year baccalaureate programs, as well as programs to promote diversity at the postdoctoral level.[6]

In closing, Valantine discussed the possibility of engaging college athletes and the NCAA to address the absence of Black men in medicine and science. Reflecting on her daughter's experience as a college athlete, Valantine said, "I started thinking about, Where is the pool? Where are all those talented Black men who through their rigorous athletic training have developed the work ethic and resilience needed for success in any field, including science? I argue that these individuals are actually under

[5] For more information on the NIH National Research Mentor Network, see https://www.nigms.nih.gov/training/dpc/pages/nrmn.aspx (accessed March 13, 2018).

[6] For more information on current programs in the National Institute of General Medical Sciences Division of Training, Workforce Development, and Diversity, including the Bridges to the Baccalaureate Program, see https://www.nigms.nih.gov/Training/Pages/TWDPrograms.aspx (accessed May 1, 2018).

the auspices of the NCAA." Valantine reported that, in 2016–2017, there were more than 55,000 NCAA Black male athletes across all divisions, of whom 21 percent reported majoring in science, technology, engineering, and mathematics fields. Additionally, Valantine found that the graduation rate among student athletes is higher than that compared with non-athlete students. Together, this suggested to her that, "There is a robust pool of Black male students able and ready to go into medical school."

HEALTH RESOURCES AND SERVICES ADMINISTRATION HEALTH WORKFORCE PRIORITIES AND PROGRAMS

Luis Padilla, M.D., FAAFP
Associate Administrator, Bureau of Health Workforce
Health Resources and Services Administration

Padilla started his talk by describing the issue of increasing representation of Black men in medicine as well aligned with the HRSA mission "to improve health and achieve health equity through access to quality services, a skilled health workforce, and innovative programs." The BHW, in particular, seeks to "improve the health of underserved and vulnerable populations by strengthening [the] health workforce and . . . connecting skilled professionals to communities in need." The BHW achieves this through three priorities: preparing a diverse workforce, improving workforce distribution, and transforming health care delivery.

The BHW administers more than 40 workforce programs, which seek to strengthen the "continuum of health profession education" from high school through service and practice. Of these, several aim to increase education and training opportunities for students and clinicians from disadvantaged backgrounds. Some examples include Area Health Education Centers (AHECs), Centers of Excellence, Health Careers Opportunity Program (HCOP), Scholarships for Disadvantaged Students, and the National Service Corps Program.[7] These programs are highly diverse. For example, more than 120,000 AHEC trainees were underrepresented minorities and 95 percent of Centers of Excellence trainees in structured programs were underrepresented minorities including 23 percent who self-identified as African American/Black. Twenty percent of HCOP grantees identify as African American, and 26 percent of those supported by the Scholarships for Disadvantaged Students identify as African American. Currently, 13 percent of the clinical workforce in the National Health Service Corps are African American men. In addition to increasing diver-

[7] For information on HRSA's BHW programs, see https://www.hrsa.gov/about/organization/bureaus/bhw/index.html (accessed March 13, 2018).

sity of the health professions, Padilla noted that these programs "also distribute that workforce across the country effectively . . . with a focus on rural and underserved [areas]."

Padilla finished his presentation by identifying potential strategies for moving forward. First, he emphasized the need to track students who participate in medical education pipeline programs. He argued, "We know that pool of applicants is out there. We just do not know what happens to them as they are going through that pipeline. . . . We need to know that the investments we have put into these programs are effective." He added that positive outcomes would include entering the health professions, especially primary care, and furthermore, whether program graduates practice in rural and underserved areas. HRSA is building a tool to track alumni of the National Service Corps using the National Practitioner Identifier. Second, Padilla outlined the BHW's focus going forward on community-based training and longitudinal training.

DISCUSSION

Valerie Montgomery Rice, M.D.,[8] concurred with Padilla about the importance of tracking and monitoring students to "understand the impact of all these persons that you have funded." She described an ongoing effort at Morehouse School of Medicine to develop an Email for Life granted to each student who comes through their National Pipeline Initiative. Morehouse would use this email to give students a career assessment from a young age, as early as middle school, and, with permission, Morehouse would reach out to students each quarter via their Email for Life. Montgomery Rice described, "You really are just teasing them every quarter, but they stay in contact. We can really build a network with that." In addition, Morehouse would build a national curriculum to pair each career goal with the necessary competences and coursework, such that "when you do these career assessment tests, you know what a kid ought to be doing based on the national standards for K through 12." In response, Padilla offered that HRSA is looking at piloting efforts to track and monitor students to lessen the work for individual universities and colleges, and proposed continuing a dialogue with Montgomery Rice.

[8] Montgomery Rice is president and dean of the Morehouse School of Medicine.

11

Reflections on the Workshop and Final Thoughts

Highlights Presented by Individual Speakers

- The cultivation of comprehensive wraparound programs that address the socioemotional circumstances around Black boys and men from childhood through graduate education are an important strategy to increase the representation of Black men in medicine. (Powell)
- Rigorous pipeline programs that start early and groom children over time are an important strategy to address the dearth of Black males in medicine. (Holden)
- Strengthening the medical education pipeline for Black men will require analytics, data, metrics, and an evidence base of effective strategies. (Reede)
- Leadership is crucial for health professional schools to address the crisis of Black men in medicine and to holding these schools accountable for increasing diversity. (Pinn)
- Acknowledging and addressing non-education-related costs of pursuing a medical education is key to addressing financial barriers in medical education. (Corbin)
- Evaluating pipeline programs is critical, but discussion is needed on what exactly should be evaluated and whether and how evaluations could or should be standardized. (Ofili)
- The opportunities for broader partnerships beyond the traditional ones are worth exploring. (Ofili)

The final session offered reflections on the workshop and an open audience discussion focused on brainstorming potential strategies to address the crisis of Black men in medicine. To launch the discussion, the moderators invited a representative from each panel—moderator or panelist—to present key points made by individual participants in their panel session. Moderator Vivian Pinn, M.D.,[1] also asked each representative to identify what they perceived to be the most important strategy from their panel to address the absence of Black men in medicine and science. Following these reflections, the moderators opened the floor for a general discussion of ideas and innovative solutions to address the crisis of Black men in medicine worth exploring. Cedric M. Bright, M.D., FACP, and Kendall Campbell, M.D., FAAFP, also moderated the discussion.[2]

REFLECTIONS ON THE WORKSHOP

Exploring Challenges and Barriers for Black Men Along the Life Trajectory

Wizdom Powell, Ph.D.,[3] framed this session as a discussion of "all of the things that happened outside of the educational system" and of the "social and lived experiences that can impact the trajectory." Powell then presented her notable points from each of the three panelists. She described how Camara Jones, M.D., M.P.H., Ph.D.,[4] identified racism as a fundamental root cause of the absence of Black men in medicine and science. She stated that addressing the challenges that Black men face will require naming, defining, and discussing levels of racism (institutional, personally mediated, and internalized). In so doing, it then becomes possible to disarm racism at each level. Jones added that it is important to ask "How is racism operating here?"

She also encouraged a change of focus from the individual to the community, to cast aside ahistorical accounts of disadvantage and debunk the myth of meritocracy, and to develop and exercise agency to set up more equitable structures. Targets for interventions Jones identified include

[1] Pinn is senior scientist emerita at the Fogarty International Center and former director (retired) in the Office of Research on Women's Health at the National Institutes of Health.

[2] Bright is associate dean for inclusive excellence, director of the Office of Special Programs, and associate professor of Medicine at the University of North Carolina School of Medicine; Campbell is associate dean for diversity and inclusion and director of the Research Group for Underrepresented Minorities in Academic Medicine at East Carolina University Brody School of Medicine.

[3] Powell is director of the Health Disparities Institute at University of Connecticut Health.

[4] Jones is senior fellow at the Satcher Health Leadership Institute at Morehouse School of Medicine.

shorter and more flexible pipelines, more seats for Black medical students, vigorous investment in public education, affordability of medical education, composition of medical school admissions committees, and practices of medical school admission committees.

Reflecting on his experience traversing the medical education pipeline, Roger A. Mitchell, Jr., M.D.,[5] discussed the need to acknowledge the "heavy backpack" young Black men carry, to act to improve the social determinants of health around some Black men, and to increase access and exposure to science, technology, engineering, and mathematics (STEM) education. In particular, Mitchell highlighted the importance of active mentoring and having a "mirror of relevance" to help young Black men develop a positive self-narrative.

In the third presentation from the panel, Arthur C. Evans, Ph.D.,[6] discussed substance use and behavioral and mental health issues as challenges to Black men's educational attainment. Specific opportunities Evans identified to potentially address these challenges include

- Disrupting the school-to-prison pipeline by identifying the youth who are experiencing social, emotional, and behavioral problems and connecting them to appropriate services;
- Making early intervention opportunities like trauma response teams and psychological first aid available at the community level without normalizing traumatic events; and
- Reframing substance use and mental health issues as mental wellness issues.

Evans also suggested celebrating resilience and focusing on strengths to develop a positive racial identity.

In summation, Powell identified the most important strategy to address challenges along the life trajectory to be the "cultivation of more comprehensive wraparound programs for Black men as they matriculate through medical education, but also before there." She continued, "We have to speak to the wounds that exist within Black men if we are going to really help them progress in the field of medicine."

[5] Mitchell is chief medical examiner for the District of Columbia.
[6] Evans is chief executive officer of the American Psychological Association.

Examining Challenges and Barriers for Black Men Along the Educational Trajectory

Lynne Holden, M.D.,[7] identified, in her view, five key points from the session on challenges and barriers for Black men along the medical education pipeline. First, she described the importance of pipeline programs and listed critical elements of these programs, for example, "K through 12 . . . longitudinal, desiloed, innovative, . . . comprehensive, involving parents, . . . mentoring, and broad community partnerships, and also incorporating protective practices for young males." Second, she discussed opportunities to expand existing programs and to look at "low hanging fruit." Some of these "low hanging fruit" might include

- Building capacity for guidance counselors and pre-health advisers,
- Finding students who take the Medical College Admission Test and do not apply to medical school,
- Finding students who are not initially accepted into a program and do not reapply,
- Reaching out to community college students,
- Expanding seats within and creating new medical schools at Historically Black Colleges and Universities (HBCUs), and
- Looking at osteopathic and offshore medical schools for lessons on increasing diversity.

Third, Holden identified the need to look at all levels of academia, especially after medical school. Specific areas for further research might include the transition between medical school and residency, especially among medical students who do not match with a residency program, or the effect of minority tax among faculty who are underrepresented minorities.[8] Fourth, she described the need for more granular data and research to correct misinformation about Black men's achievement. Fifth, Holden described the importance of leadership to address the crisis of Black men in medicine, describing how top-down efforts to increase diversity, where leadership makes a call to action and integrates equity/representation, diversity, and inclusion into their mission and vision, have been key to successfully increasing representation of underrepresented minorities. Finally, Holden identified rigorous pipeline programs that start early and

[7] Holden is president and chief executive officer of Mentoring in Medicine, emergency department physician and residency site director of the Emergency Medicine Residency Program at Montefiore Medical Center, and associate professor of clinical emergency medicine at the Albert Einstein College of Medicine.

[8] For more information on the minority tax, see Chapters 2 and 4.

groom children over time to be the most important strategy from her session to address the dearth of Black men in medicine.

Discussion on Current Innovative and Exploratory Strategies to Support Entry into Science and Medicine for Black Men

Joan Y. Reede, M.D., M.S., M.P.H., M.B.A.,[9] discussed what she perceived as several key themes across the panel session on current strategies to support Black men's entry into science and medicine. First, she pointed to investment in innovative strategies that are financially stable; follow students across a trajectory; are targeted, purposeful, and "aggressive"; and are holistic—or, have financial and leadership support, in addition to pipeline programming. Second, Reede discussed the need to focus on persistence as well as resilience. As James L. Moore III, Ph.D.,[10] described during his presentation, whereas resilience refers to bouncing back from a setback, persistence is a sustained effort. Third, Reede identified the importance of building community and socially supportive environments in which pipeline programs are embedded. Fourth, she discussed the need to address challenges in the public education system, especially the negative consequences of funding schools through local property taxes. Finally, Reede underscored the importance of data and evidence to inform program development and the need to monitor student performance and evaluate programs to ensure that programs are effective. She identified the need for analytics, data, metrics, and developing the evidence base as the most important strategies, in her opinion, from her panel session.

Exploring Accountability in Medicine and What Health Professional Schools Can Do to Address the Crisis

David Acosta, M.D.,[11] presented his notable points from the panel session on how health professional education programs can address the crisis of Black men in medicine and how they can hold themselves accountable for increasing diversity. He pointed out that leadership matters and added, "Leaders have to be deliberate and intentional about diversifying their workforce." He also questioned how schools could leverage existing leadership. He discussed accountability and connections between

[9] Reede is dean for diversity and community partnership at Harvard Medical School.

[10] Moore is interim vice provost for diversity and inclusion and chief diversity officer, executive director, Todd A. Bell National Resource Center on the African American Male, and College of Education and Human Ecology distinguished professor of urban education at The Ohio State University.

[11] Acosta is chief diversity and inclusion officer at the Association of American Medical Colleges.

actual and expected performance, asking, "How do we take ownership for becoming institutionally effective for our students' success and how to be held accountable to that?"

As a positive example of internal accountability, he pointed to the University of Illinois College of Medicine program that Dimitri T. Azar, M.D., M.B.A., dean of the college, described to cover loan and interest costs for the year following medical school graduation for students who do not match with a residency while they work to reapply and match.[12] Acosta described this approach as investing in a student's success. He also identified collaborations with other partners, including the biomedical sciences, engineered technology, and industry, and leveraging accreditation standards and elements as key strategies. As moderator, Pinn commented that what she heard as the most important strategy from this panel session was clearly the importance of leadership. She said, "Leadership from the top makes a difference of what happens underneath."

Discussion on Financial Barriers to Medical Education

Theodore Corbin, M.D., M.P.P.,[13] identified the key points, in his mind, from the panel on financial barriers. First, he endorsed increasing awareness and access to existing scholarships and other funding opportunities—including, for example, the National Medical Fellowships Emergency Scholarship Program that finances non-educational costs for students at risk of discontinuing their medical education owing to financial crises.[14]

Relatedly, he discussed the need to recognize and understand the financial challenges to preparing and applying for undergraduate education, medical school, and residency, and for required exams in addition to the costs of the education tuition, as well as the need to recognize social and familial challenges of students while in school. As additional key strategies to address financial barriers, Corbin also identified advocacy to support U.S.-born Black men in private and public institutions and exploring partnership opportunities for scholarships, endowments, and philanthropy with local efforts. He highlighted Joseph B. Hill's[15]

---

[12] For more information on this University of Illinois College of Medicine program, see Chapter 7.

[13] Corbin is vice chair for research and associate professor in the Department of Emergency Medicine at the Drexel University College of Medicine.

[14] For more information on the National Medical Fellowships Emergency Scholarship Program, see Chapter 8.

[15] Hill is senior vice president and diversity officer, Enterprise Office of Diversity, Inclusion, and Community Engagement at Thomas Jefferson University and Jefferson Health System.

presentation on the Jackson/Minton Scholarship Fund, a partnership between Thomas Jefferson University and the Sigma Pi Phi fraternity as an example. Corbin also identified what he perceived to be important gaps in the conversation—opportunities around faculty and loan repayment programs. Finally, in Corbin's view, the most important strategy to address financial barriers is acknowledging and addressing non-education-related costs of pursuing a medical education, or, "recognizing and understanding the costs that are associated with every test through every walk of life."

Examining Approaches from Philanthropy and What Philanthropies Can Do to Address the Crisis

Bright presented his highlights from the panel on philanthropy. He first commented on what he identified as themes across the panelists. Bright noted that funding programs are in place, but potential grantees need a repository to find funding opportunities and how to apply for them. He added that funding strategies at touch points along the continuum of medical education and not just at the graduate level are important. Bright also commented on the need for funders to understand the financial and social obligations that negatively affect men of color along the medical education trajectory, and proposed that many factors, including barriers to education but also social and behavioral issues, need to be addressed. To that end, programs may need some degree of flexibility to meet the varied needs of students. Finally, Bright remarked that developing strategies for sustainable financing will require thinking outside of the box.

Next, Bright offered two solutions for philanthropy to help address the shortage of Black men in medicine. First, he proposed maintaining an open dialogue between academia and philanthropies to align goals to address junctures in the medical education pipeline where Black boys and men are "leaking out." Second, he suggested the need for programs designed to help mitigate the financial and social barriers faced by under-resourced men of color. As the most important strategy from the panel, Bright identified the "need to have more committed folks that are doing these types of programs to make sure that we have the entities in place to help our students."

Discussion on Approaches in Government and What Government Can Do to Address the Crisis

Elizabeth Ofili, M.D.,[16] discussed the significant points made by the panel on government. First, she reviewed lessons from National Institutes of Health diversity initiatives, which showed that outcomes may be better than expected, it is important to know what is being measured and to understand the return on investment from these initiatives, the need for more evaluations, and a need for sustained dissemination of lessons learned. She raised the potential opportunity to partner with the National Collegiate Athletic Association (NCAA), as Hannah A. Valantine, M.D., M.R.C.P.,[17] proposed. Ofili also reviewed the effectiveness of the Health Resources and Services Administration health workforce programs at achieving a high number of trainees from historically disadvantaged backgrounds. Ofili discussed the need for long-term tracking and monitoring and to develop linkages between these tracking/monitoring systems and community-based outcomes, such as opportunities for geocoding and predictive analytics. Ofili identified the importance of evaluations and partnerships as key strategies from government. Regarding evaluations, she discussed the need to determine what exactly should be evaluated and to explore whether and how evaluations could or should be standardized. In terms of partnerships, Ofili emphasized the opportunity for broader partnerships beyond the traditional ones.

Discussion

Before moving into the open audience discussion, Pinn asked if there were any issues not discussed during the meeting that should have been. Britt raised the importance of new partners and the need to identify and recruit additional stakeholders to join the discussion. As potential stakeholder voices not well represented at the meeting, Bright offered that medical students join the discussion. Cato T. Laurencin, M.D., Ph.D.,[18] suggested that industry participate.

---

[16] Ofili is professor of medicine, director of the Clinical Research Center, and senior associate dean of Clinical and Translational Research at Morehouse School of Medicine.

[17] Valantine is chief officer, Scientific Workforce Diversity, and senior investigator at the National Heart, Lung, and Blood Institute.

[18] Laurencin is university professor, Van Dusen Distinguished Professor of Orthopaedic Surgery, and director, The Raymond and Beverly Sackler Center at the University of Connecticut.

GENERAL DISCUSSION ON INNOVATIVE SOLUTIONS AND FINAL THOUGHTS

Laurencin prompted meeting participants to generate ideas based on workshop presentations and discussion that could potentially stimulate action to address the absence of Black men in science and medicine. Note that individual participants raised the ideas presented in the following section during the discussion; in some cases, the ideas are attributed to individual speakers identified in parentheses. The ideas are not intended to reflect a consensus among workshop participants.

Strengthening the Medical Educational Pipeline

Some strategies to support individual students to navigate the medical educational pipeline include exploring, replicating, or expanding pipeline programs with potential; identifying and recruiting new and more students; and enhancing advising and mentorship for underrepresented minority students in the health professions. Specific examples of pipeline programs with potential that several participants raised include

- Creating "Persistence, Resilience, Emotional Quotient, and Perseverance" Programs for children from kindergarten through 12th grade (K–12) through college (Laurencin)
- Replicating or adapting, and scaling up, successful pipeline programs, such as those at The Ohio State University[19] and Wayne State University[20] (Laurencin)
- Increasing awareness about and access to existing programs such as through building up and enhancing a national clearinghouse of pipeline programs[21] (Valerie Montgomery Rice, M.D.,[22] and an unidentified workshop participant)
- Reviving the National Achievement Scholar program (Laurencin)
- Exploring partnerships with NCAA[23] (Laurencin)

Some participants proposed strategies that could help build up the pool of students pursuing careers in the health professions. Examples of these strategies include

---

[19] For discussion of programs at The Ohio State University, see Chapter 5.

[20] For discussion of the Wayne State University pipeline programs, see Chapter 6.

[21] For discussion of the National Clearinghouse of Pipeline Programs at Morehouse School of Medicine, see Chapter 6.

[22] Montgomery Rice is president and dean of the Morehouse School of Medicine.

[23] For discussion of the possibility of engaging college student athletes and the NCAA, see Chapter 10.

- Using sports as an entry point to attract younger children to and to engage them in medicine and science (Pinn)
- Finding and engaging talented students not already in science and medicine, such as those who excel in music (unidentified workshop participant)
- Identifying strategies to identify and support college students and graduates who do not get accepted to or do not matriculate into medical schools (e.g., funneling into postbaccalaureate programs, encouraging them to reapply) (Corbin)

Several participants also discussed the need for better advising to help students navigate STEM education and careers. Potential ideas include

- Appointing a point person in schools tasked with advising Black male students about careers in science and medicine (Pinn)
- Reaching out to college guidance counselors and pre-medicine counselors to provide better information about pursuing science and medicine careers and to correct misinformation (Pinn)
- Changing attitudes and beliefs about what obstacles to becoming doctors or researchers can and cannot be overcome (Bright)
- Engaging current students—undergraduate pre-health and science majors, medical students, and medical residents—in peer-to-peer counseling and in mentoring for younger students (e.g., K–12) (unidentified pre-health student participant)

Two additional proposed strategies that could be explored to strengthen the medical education pipeline were engaging with diversity offices (Campbell) and supporting HBCUs (unidentified workshop participant).

Engaging Organizations in Implementing Change

Some participants also raised the idea of the potential of interventions at the level of schools and organizations. These include getting academic leadership to acknowledge the absence of Black men in science and medicine as a problem and to make commitments to address the problem, harnessing technology to overcome financial barriers, and engaging with new and additional partners. In terms of gaining commitments from academic leadership, Laurencin, Montgomery Rice, and Pinn endorsed reaching out to the Association of American Medical Colleges and its Council of Deans and asking them to acknowledge the lack of Black men in medicine as a problem and making a commitment to work to change it, such as through a letter of commitment. A participant also proposed reaching out to the

American Association of Colleges of Osteopathic Medicine for a similar letter from osteopathic medical schools. With respect to technologies that colleges and universities can employ to address financial barriers associated with medical education, Pinn proposed using virtual interviews to reduce travel-associated costs, and Bright raised the potential of online resources such as the Khan Academy to prepare students for coursework and standardized tests. Many participants endorsed engaging new and additional partners, including stakeholders not represented at the meeting. Some potential partners discussed include

- Government at the national, state, and local levels, especially departments of education;
- Industry from a range of sectors, such as the biomedical sciences, pharmaceuticals, medical devices, and technology;
- Health systems and medical centers, including academic health centers through the Association of Academic Health Centers; and
- Higher education organizations like the College Board and the Association of Governing Boards of Colleges and Universities.

Engaging Communities in Implementing Change

Several participants mentioned the need for strategies to increase awareness about the absence of Black men in medicine as a problem in the community. Pinn raised the idea of developing a media and marketing strategy and increasing media outreach to reach potential students, and a participant suggested developing a marketing campaign to engage leaders (especially athletes) to speak actively about the need for Black men in medicine and the importance of this issue. Montgomery Rice also proposed identifying and recruiting technology and media partners to help develop and disseminate a communications strategy. Building on Montgomery Rice's suggestion, Azar put forward engaging Google in marketing.

Two participants raised the need to change attitudes of and expectations for the kinds of students health professional schools are looking to capture and redefining metrics of success. An unidentified participant said,

> We can be broad, and we can bring in people who medical schools cannot consider because they have not started thinking about grades and things of that nature. We can funnel them down to that space where they are ready for undergraduate; they are ready for medical school. But what that means is we have to be prepared that at the top of that funnel, there are going to be kids who are struggling. The outcomes are going to look

> different. . . . We have to have an appetite for that. We have to be okay with that.

Bright also stated,

> We have to be very cautious to make sure that we do not judge them when they walk in because of how they look or how they speak. . . . We have to be able to encourage them to continue to grow and meet them where they are as opposed to expecting them to meet us where we are.

A

Workshop Agenda

November 20–21, 2017
The Growing Absence of Black Men in Medicine
and Science: An American Crisis

WORKSHOP AGENDA

Lecture Room
2101 Constitution Avenue, NW, Washington, DC 20418

WORKSHOP OBJECTIVES

The workshop is intended to facilitate dialogue and stimulate action to increase the number of African American males in medicine. Speakers, discussants, and all participants will

1. Briefly review the past and current history of Black men in medicine and science and the challenges encountered in the transition points to becoming successful physicians and scientists.
2. Explore innovative strategies to support entry and successful passage through educational and career transition points leading to an increase in Black men in science and medicine.
3. Consider the role of government, educational systems, philanthropy, industry, and others in effecting change along educational transition points.
4. Explore ways in which innovative strategies can be shared with others, spread, and scaled up.

November 20, 2017 (Day 1)

7:30–8:30 am	**Breakfast available in East Court**
8:30–8:45 am	**Welcome and Opening Remarks** *J. Michael McGinnis, M.D., M.P.P., Leonard D. Schaeffer Executive Officer and National Academy of Medicine Senior Scholar, National Academy of Medicine* *Victor J. Dzau, M.D., President, National Academy of Medicine (video)* *Cato T. Laurencin, M.D., Ph.D., University Professor; Van Dusen Distinguished Professor of Orthopaedic Surgery; Director, The Raymond and Beverly Sackler Center, University of Connecticut*
8:45–10:00 am	**Keynote Speakers** **Moderator:** *George C. Hill, Ph.D., Levi Watkins Jr., M.D. Professor Emeritus in Medical Education; Distinguished Professor Emeritus in the Department of Pathology, Microbiology and Immunology; and Past Vice Chancellor for Equity, Diversity, and Inclusion and Chief Diversity Officer, Vanderbilt University* ***Opening Keynote*** *Louis Sullivan, M.D., Chairman and Chief Executive Officer of The Sullivan Alliance to Transform the Health Professions, and President Emeritus, Morehouse School of Medicine* ***Keynote*** *Darrell G. Kirch, M.D., President and CEO, Association of American Medical Colleges*
10:00–10:15 am	**Break**
10:15 am–12:00 pm	**Introducing Panels** *Randall C. Morgan, Jr., M.D., M.B.A., Executive Director, W. Montague Cobb/NMA Health Institute* **Panel 1: Exploring the Challenges and Barriers for Black Men Along the Life Trajectory** **Moderator:** *Wizdom Powell, Ph.D., Director, Health Disparities Institute, UConn Health*

Camara Jones, M.D., M.P.H., Ph.D., Senior Fellow, Satcher Health Leadership Institute, Morehouse School of Medicine

Roger Mitchell, Jr., M.D., Chief Medical Examiner, District of Columbia

Arthur C. Evans, Jr., Ph.D., CEO, American Psychological Association

12:00–1:00 pm **Networking Lunch: Further Discussion of Opening Talks and Panel 1**

1:00–2:30 pm **Panel 2: Exploring the Challenges and Barriers for Black Men Along the Educational Trajectory**
Moderator: *Marc Nivet, Ed.D., M.B.A., Executive Vice President for Institutional Advancement, UT Southwestern Medical Center*

Lynne Holden, M.D., President and CEO, Mentoring in Medicine, and Associate Professor of Clinical Emergency Medicine, Albert Einstein College of Medicine

Walter J. Lanier, J.D., Director of Multicultural Affairs and Community Engagement, Milwaukee Area Technical College; Alternative Campaign for Black Male Achievement, Milwaukee

C. Reynold Verret, Ph.D., President, Xavier University of Louisiana

L. D. Britt, M.D., Henry Ford Professor and Edward J. Brickhouse Chairman, Eastern Virginia Medical School

2:30–2:45 pm **Networking Break**

2:45–4:15 pm **Panel 3: Current Innovative and Exploratory Strategies to Support Entry into Science and Medicine for Black Men**
Moderator: *Freeman A. Hrabowski III, Ph.D., President, University of Maryland, Baltimore County*

André L. Churchwell, M.D., Levi Watkins Jr., M.D. Chair, Chief Diversity Officer, Vanderbilt University Medical Center; Senior Associate Dean for Diversity Affairs, Vanderbilt University School of Medicine

James L. Moore III, Ph.D., Interim Vice Provost for Diversity and Inclusion and Chief Diversity Officer, Executive Director for Todd A. Bell National Resource Center on the African American Male, and College of Education and Human Ecology Distinguished Professor of Urban Education, The Ohio State University

Marja Hurley, M.D., Professor of Medicine and Orthopedics, Associate Dean, Department of Health Career Opportunity Programs, UConn School of Medicine

Joan Y. Reede, M.D., M.S., M.P.H., M.B.A., Dean for Diversity and Community Partnership, Harvard Medical School

4:15–5:30 pm **Closing Remarks and Reflections on the Day**
Moderator: *David Satcher, M.D., Ph.D., Founding Director and Senior Advisor, Satcher Health Leadership Institute, Morehouse School of Medicine, 16th U.S. Surgeon General*[1]

Valerie Montgomery Rice, M.D., President and Dean, Morehouse School of Medicine

Wayne A. I. Frederick, M.D., M.B.A., FACS, President, Howard University

Veronica Mallett, M.D., M.M.M., Dean, School of Medicine, Meharry Medical College

Deborah Prothrow-Stith, M.D., Dean, College of Medicine, Charles R. Drew University

5:30–7:00 pm **Adjourn to Reception and Poster Session**
Poster Session: Innovative Approaches to Black Men in Medicine (Student Perspectives)

[1] David Satcher was unable to attend the meeting. L. D. Britt, M.D., Henry Ford Professor and Edward J. Brickhouse Chairman, Eastern Virginia Medical School, served as moderator for this panel in his absence.

Ross McMillan, Johns Hopkins University School of Medicine

Gabriel Felix, Howard University College of Medicine

Robert Wardlow, Johns Hopkins University School of Medicine

Abbas Rattani, Stritch School of Medicine Loyola University Chicago

Martin Campbell, Morehouse School of Medicine

November 21, 2017 (Day 2)

8:15–8:30 am

Welcome and Quick Summary of Previous Day's Discussion and Outline of the Morning Session. Introduction of Second Day Opening Speaker.
Cato T. Laurencin, M.D., Ph.D., University Professor; Van Dusen Distinguished Professor of Orthopaedic Surgery; Director, The Raymond and Beverly Sackler Center, University of Connecticut

Remarks and Reflections on the Growing Absence of Black Men in Medicine and Science
Benjamin S. Carson, Sr., M.D., Secretary, U.S. Department of Housing and Urban Development

8:30–10:00 am

Panel 4: Accountability in Medicine: What Can We Do to Address the Crisis?
Moderator: *David A. Acosta, M.D., Chief Diversity and Inclusion Officer, Association of American Medical Colleges*

M. Roy Wilson, M.D., President, Wayne State University

Dimitri T. Azar, M.D., M.B.A., Dean, University of Illinois College of Medicine

William Owen, M.D., FACP, Dean and Chancellor, Ross University School of Medicine

Adrienne White-Faines, M.P.A., FACHE, Chief Executive Officer, American Osteopathic Association

Veronica Catanese, M.D., M.B.A., Co-Secretary, Liaison Committee on Medical Education

10:00–10:15 am **Break**

10:15–11:00 am **Panel 5: Financial Barriers to Medical Education**
Moderator: *Theodore Corbin, M.D., M.P.P., Vice Chair for Research, Associate Professor, Department of Emergency Medicine, Drexel University College of Medicine*

Esther R. Dyer, M.L.S., D.L.S., President and CEO, National Medical Fellowships

Joseph B. Hill, Senior Vice President and Diversity Officer, Enterprise Office of Diversity, Inclusion & Community Engagement, Thomas Jefferson University and Jefferson Health and Alpha Boulé

Michael Knight, M.D., M.S.H.P., Assistant Professor of Medicine and Patient Safety Officer, The George Washington University; former President, Student National Medical Association

11:00 am–12:00 pm **Panel 6: Philanthropy Panel: What Can We Do to Address the Crisis?**
Moderator: *Garth Graham, M.D., Aetna Foundation*[2]

David Blumenthal, M.D., M.P.P., President, The Commonwealth Fund

John Lumpkin, M.D., Senior Vice President, Robert Wood Johnson Foundation

Alfred M. Mays, M.S., Program Officer, Burroughs Wellcome Fund

12:00–12:45 pm **Lunch**

---

[2] Garth Graham was unable to attend the meeting. Cedric M. Bright, M.D., associate dean for inclusive excellence, director, Office of Special Programs, associate professor of medicine, University of North Carolina School of Medicine, served as moderator for this session in his absence.

12:45–1:30 pm

Panel 7: Government Panel: What Can We Do to Address the Crisis?
Moderator: *Elizabeth Ofili, M.D., Professor of Medicine and Director & Senior Associate Dean, Clinical Research Center & Clinical and Translational Research, Morehouse School of Medicine*

Hannah Valantine, M.D., M.R.C.P., National Institutes of Health Workforce Diversity

Sohi Rastegar, Ph.D., Director of Office of Emerging Frontiers in Research and Innovation, National Science Foundation[3]

Luis Padilla, M.D., Associate Administrator, Bureau of Health Workforce, and Director, National Health Service Corps, Health Resources and Services Administration

1:30–3:00 pm

Report Out and Audience Discussion on Innovative Solutions and Next Steps
Moderators/Discussants:
Vivian Pinn, M.D., Senior Scientist Emerita, Fogarty International Center, and Former Director (Retired), Office of Research on Women's Health, National Institutes of Health

Cedric M. Bright, M.D., FACP, Associate Dean for Inclusive Excellence, Director, Office of Special Programs, Associate Professor of Medicine, University of North Carolina School of Medicine

Kendall Campbell, M.D., FAAFP, Associate Dean, Diversity & Inclusion, and Director, Research Group for Underrepresented Minorities in Academic Medicine, East Carolina University Brody School of Medicine

The moderator of each day's panels will be invited to present three to five key points made in each of their panel sessions as starting point for the discussion

---

[3] Sohi Rastegar was unable to attend the meeting.

Open Audience Discussion

Next Steps

3:00 pm **Adjourn**

B

Speaker Biographies

David A. Acosta, M.D., is Chief Diversity and Inclusion Officer, of the Association of American Medical Colleges (AAMC), where he provides strategic vision and leadership for the AAMC's diversity and inclusion activities across the medical education community, and leads the association's Diversity Policy and Programs unit. A physician of family medicine, Dr. Acosta joined the AAMC from the University of California (UC), Davis, School of Medicine where he served as senior associate dean for equity, diversity, and inclusion and associate vice chancellor for diversity and inclusion and chief diversity officer for UC Davis Health System. He previously served as the inaugural chief diversity officer at the University of Washington (UW) School of Medicine, where he established a rural health fellowship program for Tacoma Family Medicine, a residency program affiliated with the UW Department of Family Medicine.

Dr. Acosta received his bachelor's degree in biology from Loyola University and earned his medical degree from the University of California, Irvine, School of Medicine. He completed his residency training at Community Hospital of Sonoma County in Santa Rosa, California, and a faculty development fellowship at the UW Department of Family Medicine.

Dimitri T. Azar, M.D., M.B.A., is Dean of the University of Illinois College of Medicine. He holds the B.A. Field Chair in ophthalmologic research, and is Professor of Ophthalmology, Bioengineering, and Pharmacology. Dr. Azar joined the University of Illinois at Chicago, in 2006, as Head of the Department of Ophthalmology and Visual Sciences after serving as tenured Professor of Ophthalmology at Harvard Medical School, Director of the Cornea Service at the Massachusetts Eye and Ear Infirmary, Senior Scientist at the Schepens Eye Institute, and as faculty at the Johns Hopkins University School of Medicine. Dr. Azar brings experience in administration, research, education, and clinical practice to his position as Dean of the College of Medicine. He earned an executive M.B.A. with high honors from the University of Chicago. Dr. Azar is the author of more than 400 scientific articles and book chapters. He is the editor of 14 books in ophthalmology and he holds 15 patents. Dr. Azar has been named one of The Best Doctors in America and/or one of the Castle Connolly regional Top Doctors in America annually since 1994. He is a leader in basic science and clinically related vision research, making significant contributions to the treatment of corneal diseases and to advances in refractive surgery through mathematical analyses and applications of advanced optics. His basic science research on matrix metalloproteinases in corneal wound healing and angiogenesis has been continually funded by the National Eye Institute R01 award since 1993. He serves as a trustee for the Chicago Ophthalmological Society and for the Association of Research and Vision in Ophthalmology. Dr. Azar has also received multiple leadership awards, including the 2009 Lans Distinguished Award and the University of Illinois at Chicago Scholar Award.

David Blumenthal, M.D., M.P.P., is President of The Commonwealth Fund, a national philanthropy engaged in independent research on health and social policy issues. Dr. Blumenthal is formerly the Samuel O. Thier Professor of Medicine at Harvard Medical School and Chief Health Information and Innovation Officer at Partners Healthcare System in Boston. From 2009 to 2011, he served as the National Coordinator for Health Information Technology, with the charge to build an interoperable, private, and secure nationwide health information system and to support the widespread, meaningful use of health information technology. He succeeded in putting in place one of the largest publicly funded infrastructure investments the nation has ever made in such a short time period, in health care or any other field.

Previously, Dr. Blumenthal was a practicing primary care physician, director of the Institute for Health Policy, and professor of medicine and health policy at Massachusetts General Hospital/Partners Healthcare System and Harvard Medical School. He is the author of more than 250 books and scholarly publications, including most recently, *Heart of Power: Health and Politics in the Oval Office*. He is a member of the National Academy of Medicine and serves on the editorial boards of the *New England Journal of Medicine* and the *Journal of Delivery Science and Innovation*. He has also served on the staff of the U.S. Senate Subcommittee on Health and Scientific Research; is the founding chairman of AcademyHealth, the national organization of health services researchers; and is a trustee of the University of Pennsylvania Health System.

Dr. Blumenthal received his undergraduate, medical, and public policy degrees from Harvard University and completed his residency in internal medicine at Massachusetts General Hospital. With his colleagues from Harvard Medical School, he authored the seminal studies on the adoption and use of health information technology in the United States. He has held several leadership positions in medicine, government, and academia, including senior vice president at Boston's Brigham and Women's Hospital and executive director of the Center for Health Policy and Management and lecturer on public policy at the Kennedy School of Government. He served previously on the board of the University of Chicago Health System and is recipient of the Distinguished Investigator Award from AcademyHealth, an Honorary Doctor of Humane Letters from Rush University, and an Honorary Doctor of Science from Claremont Graduate University and the State University of New York Downstate.

Cedric M. Bright, M.D., FACP, is the Associate Dean for Inclusive Excellence, Director of the Office of Special Programs, and Associate Professor in the Division of General Medicine and Clinical Epidemiology at the University of North Carolina School of Medicine. He served as the 112th President of the National Medical Association from 2011 to 2012. He was previously Associate Clinical Professor of Internal Medicine and Community and Family Medicine at Duke University and a staff physician at the VA Medical Center in Durham. Dr. Bright also served on the North Carolina Medical Society Patient Safety Taskforce; chaired the board of directors at the Lincoln Community Health Center; has spoken about health disparities before the Congressional Black Caucus; was a medical ambassador to Ghana; and has served as a mentor for the Student National Medical Association. He is a dedicated leader in delivering patient equity through broader access, and is a staunch proponent of health care reform.

L. D. Britt, M.D., M.P.H., D.Sc. (Hon.), FACS, FCCM, FRCSEng (Hon.), FRCSEd (Hon.), FWACS (Hon.), FRCSI (Hon.), FCS(SA) (Hon.), a native of Suffolk, Virginia, received his B.A. with Distinction from the University of Virginia. Dr. Britt, a graduate of Harvard Medical School and Harvard School of Public Health, is the Henry Ford Professor and Edward J. Brickhouse Chairman of the Department of Surgery at Eastern Virginia Medical School. He is the author of more than 220 peer-reviewed publications, more than 50 book chapters and non-peer-reviewed articles, and three books, including a recent edition of the highly touted *Acute Care Surgery* (Lippincott, Williams & Wilkens, Medford, NJ). He serves on numerous editorial boards, including the *Annals of Surgery*, *Archives of Surgery*, *World Journal of Surgery*, *Journal of the American College of Surgeons*, the *American Journal of Surgery* (Associate Editor), the *Journal of Trauma*, *Shock*, *Journal of Surgical Education*, the *American Surgeon*, and others. In addition, he is a reviewer for the *New England Journal of Medicine*.

Dr. Britt, a member of Alpha Omega Alpha, is the recipient of the nation's highest teaching award in medicine—the Robert J. Glaser Distinguished Teaching Award, which is given by the AAMC in conjunction with Alpha Omega Alpha. He was honored by the Association of Surgical Education with its lifetime achievement award—the Distinguished Educator Award—given annually to one person considered by his peers to be a true master. More than 190 institutions throughout the world have invited him to be their distinguished visiting professor. He was recently the William P. Longmire, M.D., Visiting Professor at the University of California, Los Angeles.

Dr. Britt is the past President of the Society of Surgical Chairs and the past Chairman of the ACGME Residency Review Committee for Surgery. Also, he is past Secretary of the Southern Surgical Association, the past Recorder/Program Chair for the American Association for the Surgery of Trauma, and past President of the Southeastern Surgical Congress, the Halsted Society, and the Southern Surgical Association. Dr. Britt is the past Chairman of the Board of Regents of the American College of Surgeons. He is also past President of the American College of Surgeons, the American Association for the Surgery of Trauma, and the American Surgical Association.

At the inaugural presidential ceremony held in Washington, DC, during the 96th annual Clinical Congress of the American College of Surgeons, Dr. Britt was awarded the U.S. Surgeon General's medallion for his outstanding achievements in medicine. The Honorable Regina Benjamin, M.D., the 18th U.S. Surgeon General, presented this award at a formal ceremony. Dr. Britt was also appointed to the Robert Wood Johnson Clinical Scholar Program National Advisory Committee. The National Library of Medicine of the National Institutes of Health (in collaboration with the Reginald F. Lewis Museum of Maryland African American History and Culture) featured Dr. Britt for his contributions to academic surgery. President George W. Bush recognized Dr. Britt's leadership role in medicine and nominated him to the Board of Regents of the Uniformed Services University (confirmed by the U.S. Senate). At the end of his tenure, Dr. Britt was awarded the coveted Distinguished Service Medal. The National Board of Medical Examiners also awarded him the Edithe J. Levit Distinguished Service Award. An active participant in the community, Dr. Britt has received numerous awards for public service. Dr. Britt is the recipient of the 2010 Colgate Darden Citizen of the Year Award and the 2011 Dr. Martin Luther King, Jr., Community Award. *Atlanta Post* recently highlighted him as one of the top 21 black doctors in America. *Ebony* magazine recently listed him as one of the most influential African Americans in the nation. At the 2012 annual meeting of the American Surgical Association, Dr. Britt became the 132nd President of the organization. He was conferred an Honorary Doctorate by the President of Tuskegee University. Dr. Britt was also elected to the position of Commissioner of The Joint Commission (formerly JACHO). In 2012, he was conferred an Honorary Fellowship in the French Academy of Surgery and the Colleges of Medicine of South Africa. Having recently been awarded an Honorary Fellowship in the Royal College of Surgeons of Glasgow, Dr. Britt now has the distinction of receiving the highest honor given by each of the four Royal Colleges in the United Kingdom—England, Edinburg, Ireland, and Glasgow. Dr. Britt, author of the term *acute care surgery* and one of the principal architects of this emerging specialty, was the 2013 recipient of the prestigious Roswell Park Medal. At the 2015 annual meeting of the Society of Critical Care Medicine, Dr. Britt was bestowed the coveted title of "Master of Critical Care Medicine" by the American College of Critical Care Medicine. In 2015, Virginia Governor Terry McAuliffe appointed Dr. Britt to the Board of Visitors of the University of Virginia. Also, the Southern Surgical Association awarded Dr. Britt the organization's highest accolade—Honorary Fellowship—at its 2015 annual meeting. In the spring of 2016, Dr. Britt was awarded the Urban League of Hampton Roads Professor Marian Capps Memorial Award for his accomplishments in community service through education. At the 148th commencement at Howard University, Dr. Britt was conferred an honorary doctorate (Doctor of Science). In the summer of 2016 Dr. Britt serendipitously conducted his 200th visiting professorship at Cook County Hospital in Chicago, Illinois (where Dr. Britt completed his residency training). He was the inaugural John A. Barrett, M.D. Lecturer who kicked off the 50th anniversary celebration for the Cook County Hospital Trauma Unit. Dr. Britt was elected to the National Academy of Medicine in 2016.

Kendall M. Campbell, M.D., FAAFP, is Associate Dean for Diversity and Inclusion and Director of the Research Group for Underrepresented Minorities in Academic Medicine at the East Carolina University Brody School of Medicine. Dr. Campbell was one of the first Science Students Together Reaching Instructional Diversity and Excellence (SSTRIDE) mentors and instructors. SSTRIDE seeks to identify and encourage middle and high school students from underrepresented backgrounds, including those from rural communities. He became a part of the program in 1994 while an undergraduate student and chemistry pre-med major at

Florida A&M University. After completing his undergraduate degree, Dr. Campbell attended the Program in Medical Sciences, a 1-year program created to help promote diversity in Florida's medical schools by attracting more students from backgrounds underrepresented in medicine and in the Florida physician workforce. After the completion of medical school, he went on to become a board-certified family physician with special interests in underserved care and teaching. Dr. Campbell is the learning center advisor for the Bridge to Clinical Medicine master's degree program, a program to increase underrepresented groups in medicine, and as codirector of the Center for Underrepresented Minorities in Academic Medicine conducts research to study issues affecting underrepresented minority faculty in medical education. He sees patients at Bond Community Health Center, a community health center for the underserved.

Benjamin S. Carson, Sr., M.D., is the 17th Secretary of the U.S. Department of Housing and Urban Development. For nearly 30 years, Secretary Carson served as Director of Pediatric Neurosurgery at the Johns Hopkins Children's Center, a position he assumed when he was just 33 years old, becoming the youngest major division director in the hospital's history. In 1987, he successfully performed the first separation of craniopagus twins conjoined at the back of the head. He also performed the first fully successful separation of type-2 vertical craniopagus twins in 1997 in South Africa.

Dr. Carson received dozens of honors and awards in recognition of his achievements including the Presidential Medal of Freedom, the nation's highest civilian honor. He is also a recipient of the Spingarn Medal, the highest honor bestowed by the National Association for the Advancement of Colored People.

Dr. Carson authored nine books, four of which he co-wrote with his wife Candy. The U.S. News Media Group and Harvard's Center for Public Leadership named him among "America's Best Leaders" in 2008.

Dr. Carson and his wife cofounded the Carson Scholars Fund, which recognizes young people of all backgrounds for exceptional academic and humanitarian accomplishments. The Fund currently operates in 50 states and the District of Columbia, and has recognized more than 7,300 scholars, awarded more than $7.3 million in scholarships, and installed more than 150 Ben Carson Reading Rooms around the country.

Born in Detroit to a single mother with a 3rd-grade education who worked multiple jobs to support their family, Dr. Carson was raised to love reading and education. He graduated from Yale University and earned his M.D. from the University of Michigan Medical School.

Veronica Catanese, M.D., M.B.A., is Cosecretary of the Liaison Committee on Medical Education (LCME) and Senior Director of accreditation services at the AAMC. She leads the AAMC's accreditation services unit and collaborates with her counterpart at the American Medical Association to accredit U.S. M.D.-granting medical schools.

Dr. Catanese most recently served as Vice Dean, Dean for academic affairs, and Principal Business Officer at the Donald and Barbara Zucker School of Medicine at Hofstra Northwell, where she was the Dr. Leo A. Guthart Professor of Medicine and a member of the school's founding team. Before Hofstra Northwell, Dr. Catanese was a tenured faculty member in the departments of medicine and cell biology at New York University (NYU) School of Medicine, where she spent a decade as Senior Associate Dean for education and student affairs. During her time at Hofstra Northwell and at NYU, she participated in six LCME accreditation cycles, leading the preparations on four occasions.

Dr. Catanese has served in various leadership roles with the American Federation for Medical Research, including as a National Councilor, Public Policy Chair, President, and Foundation President, as well as Editor-in-Chief of the *Journal of Investigative Medicine*. She has chaired a National Institutes of Health (NIH) biomedical technology transfer study section, and was selected as a member of the Institute of Medicine's Clinical Research Roundtable and Cochair of the training subcommittee of the NIH Director's Clinical Research Roadmap working group.

Dr. Catanese received her bachelor's degree from Wellesley College and earned her medical degree from NYU School of Medicine, where she was elected to membership in Alpha Omega Alpha. She completed her residency and chief residency in internal medicine and a clinical fellowship in endocrinology, diabetes, and metabolism at NYU Medical Center, followed by a research fellowship at Joslin Diabetes Center. She received her M.B.A. from the NYU Stern School of Business.

André L. Churchwell, M.D., is Levi Watkins Jr., M.D. Chair and Vanderbilt University Medical Center's Chief Diversity Officer, and a Professor of Medicine (Cardiology), Professor of Radiology and Radiological Sciences, Professor of Biomedical Engineering, and Senior Associate Dean for Diversity Affairs at Vanderbilt University School of Medicine. He was named the 2005 Walter R. Murray Jr. Distinguished Alumnus by the Association of Vanderbilt Black Alumni. The award recognizes lifetime achievements in personal, professional, and community arenas.

Dr. Churchwell graduated from the Vanderbilt School of Engineering magna cum laude in 1975. He won the Biomedical Engineering Student Program Award that same year. He received his medical degree from Harvard Medical School in 1979 and later completed his internship, residency, and cardiology fellowship at Emory University School of Medicine and affiliated hospitals in Atlanta. In addition, he was the first African American chief medical resident at Grady Memorial Hospital (1984–1985).

Dr. Churchwell received the J. Willis Hurst Award for Best Clinical Teacher in 1991 from Emory, and in 2004 he was named the Emory University School of Medicine Resident Alumni Distinguished Achievement Award winner. For the past 10 years he has been named one of the nation's top cardiologists in "The Best Doctors in America."

In 1986, while at Emory, he was also named Most Outstanding House Officer, made an honorary Morehouse Medical School class member, and he received a Robert Wood Johnson Foundation Minority Medical Faculty Development Award.

In 2010, he was awarded the Distinguished Alumnus Award of Vanderbilt University School of Engineering. Along with his physician brothers Kevin and Keith, he received the 2011 Trumpet Award for Medicine.

He serves on many medical school committees including the Admission and Promotion Committees and recently was named Dean of Diversity for Undergraduate Medical Education to add to his current role in the Dean's office.

In 2012 and 2013, the Vanderbilt University Organization of Black Graduate and Professional Students honored Dr. Churchwell with one of the organization's first Distinguished Faculty Awards. He was also recognized with an American Registry Most Compassionate Doctor Award. From 2010 to 2013, he has been awarded the Professional Research Consultants' Five-Star Excellence Award—Top 10% Nationally for "Excellent" Responses for Medical Specialty Services and Overall Quality. And in 2014, he was honored as one of the Top 15 Most Influential African American Medical Educators by *Black Health Magazine*.

Furthermore, he was elected in 2012 to serve as the southern representative for the Group on Diversity and Inclusion for the AAMC. Since 2011, he has served on the editorial board of *Cardiovascular Engineering and Technology: A Journal of the Biomedical Engineering Society*. In 2013, he helped create the Hurst-Logue-Wenger Cardiovascular Fellows Society (HLWCFS) of Emory University School of Medicine and was elected the first President of HLWCFS.

Theodore Corbin, M.D., M.P.P., is Vice Chair for Research and an Associate Professor in the Department of Emergency Medicine at the Drexel University College of Medicine. He also serves as the Medical Director of the "Healing Hurt People" program, an emergency department–based, trauma-informed intervention strategy that identifies victims of intentional injury. Dr. Corbin received his master's in public policy from the Woodrow Wilson School at Princeton University. Recipient of the 2017

Drexel University College of Medicine Distinguished Alumni, Dr. Corbin also codirects the Center for Nonviolence and Social Justice at Drexel University School of Public Health, where he holds a joint appointment. He was awarded a Stoneleigh Foundation Fellowship and an Annie E. Casey Foundation grant to explore the impact of posttraumatic stress disorder on violently injured youth and young adults, and to evaluate the effectiveness of Healing Hurt People. His work focuses broadly on addressing the trauma in the lives of victims of violence, especially boys and men of color for whom violence is a leading cause of disability and death.

Esther R. Dyer, M.L.S., D.L.S., is President and Chief Executive Officer of National Medical Fellowships (NMF), a nonprofit organization dedicated to building the next generation of health care leaders. Founded in 1946, NMF has provided more than 30,000 scholarships to diverse students in medicine and the health professions. Previously, she was Executive Director of the American-Italian Cancer Foundation and the U.S. Representative of the European School of Oncology. Prior positions have included Director of Public Affairs for Empire Blue Cross/Director of the Health Services Research Fund; Executive Director of the NYC March of Dimes; External Affairs Advisor to the Center for Bioenvironmental Research at Tulane and Xavier Universities; Senior Advisor External Affairs, Columbia Cornell Cares; and Assistant Professor and Member of the Graduate Faculty at Rutgers University.

She holds a doctorate in library science, Columbia University; a Certificado del Curso Medio, Universidad de Salamanca; masters in information policy, Rockefeller College, SUNY Albany (Distinguished Alumna); and a bachelors in secondary education, SUNY, New Paltz. She serves as a Board Member of the Lower Westside Home Health Agency, the Circumnavigators Club Foundation, and the Emy and Emil Herzfeld Foundation. She is a Life Member of the Circumnavigator's Club and International President (2010–2012).

Victor J. Dzau, M.D., is the President of the National Academy of Medicine (NAM), formerly the Institute of Medicine (IOM). In addition, he serves as Chair of the Health and Medicine Division Committee of the National Academies of Sciences, Engineering, and Medicine. He is Chancellor Emeritus and James B. Duke Professor of Medicine at Duke University and the past President and Chief Executive Officer of the Duke University Health System. Previously, Dr. Dzau was the Hersey Professor of Theory and Practice of Medicine and Chairman of Medicine at Harvard Medical School's Brigham and Women's Hospital, as well as Chairman of the Department of Medicine at Stanford University.

Dr. Dzau has made a significant impact on medicine through his research in cardiovascular medicine and genetics, his pioneering of the discipline of vascular medicine, and his leadership in health care innovation. His important work on the renin angiotensin system (RAS) paved the way for the contemporary understanding of RAS in cardiovascular disease and the development of RAS inhibitors as widely used lifesaving drugs. Dr. Dzau also pioneered gene therapy for vascular disease, and his recent work on stem cell paracrine mechanisms and the use of microRNA in direct reprogramming provides novel insight into stem cell biology and regenerative medicine.

In his role as a leader in health care, Dr. Dzau has led efforts in health care innovation. His vision is for academic health sciences centers to lead the transformation of medicine through innovation, translation, and globalization. Leading this vision at Duke, he and his colleagues developed the Duke Translational Medicine Institute, the Duke Global Health Institute, the Duke-National University of Singapore Graduate Medical School, and the Duke Institute for Health Innovation. These initiatives create a seamless continuum from discovery and translational sciences to clinical care, and they promote transformative innovation in health.

As one of the world's preeminent academic health leaders, Dr. Dzau advises governments, corporations, and universities worldwide. He has been a member of the Council of the IOM and the Advisory Committee to the Director of the NIH, as well as Chair of the NIH Cardiovascular Disease Advisory Committee and the Association of Academic Health Centers. He served on the Governing Board of the Duke-National University of Singapore Graduate Medical School and the Board of Health Governors of the World Economic Forum and chaired its Global Agenda Council on Personalized and Precision Medicine. He also served as the Senior Health Policy Advisor to Her Highness Sheikha Moza (Chair of the Qatar Foundation). Currently, he is a member of the Board of Directors of the Singapore Health System, the Expert Board of the Imperial College Health Partners, UK, and the International Advisory Board of the Biomedical Science Council of Singapore. In 2011, he led a partnership between Duke University, the World Economic Forum, and McKinsey, and he founded the International Partnership for Innovative Healthcare Delivery and currently chairs its Board of Directors.

Among his honors and recognitions are the Gustav Nylin Medal from the Swedish Royal College of Medicine; the Max Delbruck Medal from Humboldt University, Charité, and the Max Planck Institute; the Commemorative Gold Medal from the Ludwig Maximilian University of Munich; the Inaugural Hatter Award from the Medical Research Council of South Africa; the Polzer Prize from the European Academy of Sciences and Arts; the Novartis Award for Hypertension Research; the Distinguished Scientist Award from the American Heart Association (AHA);

and the AHA Research Achievement Award for his contributions to cardiovascular biology and medicine. Recently, he was awarded the Public Service Medal by the President of Singapore. He has received 10 honorary doctorates.

Arthur C. Evans, Jr., Ph.D., is Chief Executive Officer of the American Psychological Association (APA). In this position, he heads the leading scientific and professional organization representing psychology in the United States, with nearly 115,700 researchers, educators, clinicians, consultants, and students as its members. Before joining APA, Dr. Evans spent 12 years as commissioner of Philadelphia's Department of Behavioral Health and Intellectual disAbility Service, a $1.2 billion health care agency that is the behavioral health and intellectual disabilities safety net for 1.5 million Philadelphians. He realigned the agency's treatment philosophy, service delivery models, and fiscal policies to improve health outcomes and increase the efficiency of the service system. The transformation of the Philadelphia service system has saved millions of dollars that the city reinvested in other community-based services.

Dr. Evans has been recognized nationally and internationally for his work in behavioral health care policy and service delivery innovation. In 2015, he was recognized by the White House as an "Advocate for Action" by the Office of National Drug Control Policy. In 2013, he received the American Medical Association's top government service award in health care, the Dr. Nathan Davis Award for Outstanding Government Service. Dr. Evans is also regarded as a strong mental health advocate and was recognized by Faces and Voices of Recovery with the Lisa Mojer-Torres Award. In 2017, he was awarded the Visionary Leadership Award by the National Council of Behavioral Health and inducted into the Florida Atlantic University Alumni Hall of Fame at his alma mater. He has also been recognized as a strong advocate for social justice, having received three different Martin Luther King Jr. awards.

Dr. Evans holds faculty appointments at the University of Pennsylvania Perelman School of Medicine, Drexel University School of Public Health, and the Philadelphia College of Osteopathic Medicine, and he has held a faculty appointment at the Yale University School of Medicine.

Earlier in his career, Dr. Evans was deputy commissioner of the Connecticut Department of Mental Health & Addiction Services, where he led major strategic initiatives in the state's behavioral health care system. Similar to his work in Philadelphia, he was instrumental in implementing a recovery-oriented policy framework, addressing health care disparities, increasing the use of evidence-based practices, and significantly improving community engagement. He also developed a thriving private practice.

Dr. Evans is the author or coauthor of 40 peer-reviewed research articles and of numerous chapters, reviews, and editorials. He is a member of the editorial board of the *Journal of Substance Abuse Treatment* and a fellow and member of the board of trustees of the College of Physicians of Philadelphia.

Wayne A. I. Frederick, M.D., M.B.A., FACS, is Howard University's 17th president. His goal is to enhance the Howard University legacy, ensure that the University maximizes its impact, and that its students receive a well-rounded educational experience.

As an undergraduate student, Frederick was admitted to Howard's rigorous B.S./M.D. dual degree program. He completed the requirements for both the B.S. and M.D. degree in 6 years, allowing him to earn both degrees by the age of 22. He also received a master of business administration degree from Howard University's School of Business in 2011.

Dr. Frederick continues to operate and lecture actively; the focal point of his medical research is to narrow the disparity in all cancer-care outcomes, with a focus on gastrointestinal cancers. A distinguished researcher and surgeon, Dr. Frederick has also received various awards honoring his scholarship and service.

In January 2017, the Federal Reserve System Board of Governors elected Dr. Frederick to the Federal Reserve Bank of Richmond's Baltimore Branch, and in May 2016, President Barack H. Obama elected Dr. Frederick to the Board of Advisors for the White House Initiative on Historically Black Colleges and Universities (HBCUs). In April 2016, Dr. Frederick became a member of the American Surgical Association, known as the nation's oldest and most prestigious surgical organization.

Garth Graham, M.D., M.P.H., FACP, FACC,[1] is a leading authority on social determinants of health. President of the Aetna Foundation and Vice President of Community Health for Aetna Inc., he is also a cardiologist and public health expert.

Dr. Graham oversees the community health initiatives for the Foundation and Aetna Inc., bringing his experience as a former deputy assistant secretary at the U.S. Department of Health and Human Services under the Obama and Bush administrations where he also ran the Office of Minority Health. He directed the development of the federal government's first National Health Disparities Plan released under the Obama administration.

Dr. Graham has been a contributor to *The Hill*, the *Chicago Tribune*, *Fortune*, *Quartz*, *Health Affairs*, and *Ebony*, and has been featured in *Essence*,

[1] Garth Graham was unable to attend the meeting.

CNN, and *The New York Times* among others. His original research has been published in the *Journal of the American Medical Association, American Journal of Public Health, Health Affairs*, and other publications. Along with his role at the Aetna Foundation, Dr. Graham is a clinical associate professor of medicine at the University of Connecticut.

Prior to joining the Foundation, in his role as the assistant dean for health policy at the University of Florida School of Medicine, Garth led several research initiatives looking at how to improve outcomes and readmission rates in cardiac patients in underserved populations. He contributes to several boards including being named by the President to the U.S. Federal Coordinating Council on Comparative Effectiveness Research; the National Academies of Sciences, Engineering, and Medicine's Roundtable on Population Health and Public Health Practice; the American Heart Association/American Stroke Association National Quality Oversight Committee; the American College of Cardiology/American Heart Association Task Force on Clinical Data Standards; and many others.

Dr. Graham holds a medical degree from Yale School of Medicine, a master's in public health from Yale School of Public Health, and a bachelor of science in biology from Florida International University in Miami. He completed clinical training in cardiology and interventional cardiology at Massachusetts General Hospital and Johns Hopkins. He holds three board certifications: internal medicine, cardiology, and interventional cardiology.

George C. Hill, Ph.D., is Levi Watkins Jr., M.D. Professor Emeritus in Medical Education and Distinguished Professor Emeritus in the Department of Pathology, Microbiology and Immunology. He was Vanderbilt University's first Vice Chancellor for Diversity, Equity and Inclusion and Chief Diversity Officer, a position he held until his retirement in July 2017. He served as Assistant Vice Chancellor for Multicultural Affairs and Special Assistant to the Provost for Health Affairs from 2011 to 2012. From 2002 to 2011, he served as the Vanderbilt University School of Medicine's first Associate Dean for Diversity in Medical Education. Under Dr. Hill's leadership, the medical school made significant progress toward increasing the diversity of the medical school class to more broadly represent different races/ethnicities, sexual orientations, economic backgrounds, religious backgrounds, and rural-vs.-urban upbringing.

Prior to being recruited to Vanderbilt in 2002, Dr. Hill spent 19 years at Meharry Medical College, where he served in a variety of senior faculty and administrative roles including dean of the School of Graduate Studies and Research, vice president for research, associate vice president for international affairs, and director of the Division of Biomedical Sciences. In 2013, he received the Levi Watkins Jr., M.D. Award from the Vanderbilt University School of Medicine for fostering diversity and inclusion throughout the university as well as nationally.

Dr. Hill has mentored and trained hundreds of Ph.D. students, M.S. students, and postdoctoral fellows. In 1999, he was recognized as a "Giant in Science" by the Quality Education for Minorities Network for his commitment to motivating minority students to pursue the sciences.

Dr. Hill has led a distinguished career in biomedical research and medical education and is a world-renowned microbiologist. His laboratory was the first to grow the infective protozoan that carries sleeping sickness. His work to characterize the protozoan gave scientists an opportunity to develop drugs to treat sleeping sickness and was published in the leading scientific journal *Science*.

A member of the National Academy of Medicine since 1998, Hill was elected a fellow of the Academy of Microbiology in 2002. In 2011, he was elected a fellow of the American Association for the Advancement of Science (AAAS) and was appointed to the NIH Fogarty International Center Scientific Advisory Board. The American Association for the Advancement of Science cited Dr. Hill's leadership as president of the National Foundation for Infectious Diseases, where he also received the organization's Utz Leadership Award, as well as his work advancing a diverse workplace and his contributions to research into tropical diseases. Dr. Hill was elected a fellow of health disparities of the Cobb Institute of the National Medical Association in 2014. He currently serves on the Cooper Medical School of Rowan University Medical Board.

Previous appointments and awards include serving as a Fulbright Scholar at the University of Nairobi and as an NIH research fellow at the University of Cambridge, Great Britain; receiving the Seymour Hunter Prize from the Society of Protozoologists; and serving on the National Institute for General Medical Sciences Council and the National Institute of Allergy and Infectious Diseases Board of Scientific Counselors.

Dr. Hill graduated from Rutgers in 1961 and went on to receive his M.S. from Howard University and his Ph.D. from New York University, where he launched his career in the biomedical sciences.

Joseph B. Hill is Senior Vice President and Chief Diversity Officer for Thomas Jefferson University and Jefferson Health System in Philadelphia, Pennsylvania. In this role, he is responsible for leading the integration of diversity, inclusion, and health equity to ensure excellence in education, research and patient care.

Prior to joining Thomas Jefferson University and Jefferson Health System in 2015, Mr. Hill served as Vice President and Chief Diversity Officer for Froedtert and the Medical College of Wisconsin in Milwaukee where he developed a diversity and inclusion program that became an integral part of the health system's values, strategy, and operational initiatives. Under his leadership, Froedtert's diversity and inclusion team was nationally recognized for supplier diversity and health care equality.

From 2007 to 2010, Mr. Hill was the Managing Director of Diversity and Inclusion for the American Cancer Society's national home office in Atlanta, Georgia, where he provided strategic direction, management, and support for diversity and inclusion initiatives. He was also the American Cancer Society's National Director of Diversity and External Partnerships with responsibility for working with all 17 divisions on diversity and inclusion strategies. In addition, he served as the senior leader in the development and implementation of business relationships with key diverse community organizations and leaders. Prior to the American Cancer Society, Mr. Hill applied his skills at the corporate headquarters of Cingular Wireless, which became AT&T Mobility, where he served as Senior Diversity Manager.

Mr. Hill earned a B.A. from Virginia Union University, an M.A. from Howard University, and a Certificate in Diversity Management in Health Care from Georgetown University and the Institute for Diversity in Health Management.

A native of Buffalo, New York, Mr. Hill is a frequent speaker at national forums where he shares his insights and experience on the importance of diversity and strategic partnerships in both the for-profit and nonprofit sectors. Mr. Hill serves as a board member for Garden and Associates, LLC and the National Football Players Father's Association, and is on the Advisory Board for Usher's New Look Foundation.

Lynne Holden, M.D., is working to change the face of medicine. She is the energetic President, Chief Executive Officer, and visionary of Mentoring in Medicine. Dr. Holden provides the overall leadership, recruits volunteers, facilitates program development, creates organizational strategy, and establishes collaborative partnerships. Dr. Holden earned her B.S. in zoology from Howard University. After graduating from Temple University School of Medicine and completing her residency in emergency medicine at the Albert Einstein College of Medicine-Jacobi/Montefiore Emergency Medicine Residency Program, she is now a practicing Emergency Department Physician at Montefiore Medical Center and serves as its Residency Site Director of the Emergency Medicine Residency Program. She is also an Associate Professor of Clinical Emergency Medicine at the Albert Einstein College of Medicine, where she cochairs the Admissions Committee.

Her many accolades and awards include

- Albert Einstein College of Medicine Leo Davidoff Society Teaching Award—2002
- Universal Sisters' Commitment to Women's Health Award—2008
- Maybelline NY-Essence Empowerment through Education Award—2007
- Society of Emergency Medicine Diversity Interest Group's first Visionary Educator Award— 2008
- Woman of the Year Award by the National Council of Negro Women, North Bronx Section—2009
- Robert Wood Johnson Foundation Community Health Leader—2009
- Washington Post Root 100 Leader—2010
- Lifetime TV *Remarkable Woman*—2010
- Featured on CNN's Sanjay Gupta's *Human Factor*—2011
- Outstanding Contribution to Health Professional Education Award from NAMME–Northeast—2008
- Paul Burgess Community Advocate Award, Harlem Health Promotion Center, Mailman School of Public Health, Columbia University—2008
- Gloria Bynoe Thomas Award by the City College Minority Association of Pre–Health Students—2009
- Rev. Cannon Stewart Community Service Award by the Harlem Congregations for Community Improvement, Inc.—2009

Freeman A. Hrabowski III, Ph.D., President of UMBC (University of Maryland, Baltimore County) since 1992, is a consultant on science and math education to national agencies, universities, and school systems. He was named by President Obama to chair the President's Advisory Commission on Educational Excellence for African Americans. He also chaired the National Academies' committee that produced the report *Expanding Underrepresented Minority Participation: America's Science and Technology Talent at the Crossroads* (2011).

Named one of the 100 Most Influential People in the World by *TIME* (2012) and one of America's Best Leaders by *U.S. News & World Report* (2008), he also received TIAA-CREF's Theodore M. Hesburgh Award for Leadership Excellence (2011), the Carnegie Corporation's Academic Leadership Award (2011), and the Heinz Award (2012) for contributions to improving the "Human Condition." UMBC has been recognized as a model for inclusive excellence by such publications as *U.S. News & World Report*, which for the past 8 years has recognized UMBC as a national leader in academic innovation and undergraduate teaching.

Marja Hurley, M.D., is Professor of Medicine and Orthopedics and Member of the Institute of Systems Genomics at the UConn School of Medicine.

She is the first woman of color to receive the doctorate of medicine from UConn School of Medicine and the first to be a tenured full professor at the UConn School of Medicine. Dr. Hurley served as interim Senior Associate Dean for Education and Academic Affairs, Chair of the Education Council, and Chair of the Committee on Undergraduate Medical Education, UConn School of Medicine. Dr. Hurley has made outstanding contributions as an administrator, educator, and research scientist at UConn Health and received local, national, and international recognition and awards for her accomplishments in several of these domains. These include recipient of the prestigious 2016 Lawrence G. Raisz Esteemed Award from the American Society of Bone Mineral Research for preclinical translational research; induction into the Connecticut Academy of Science and Engineering; UConn Health Board of Directors Faculty Recognition Award; and the Neag Medal of Honor. She also received the University of Connecticut's first Martin Luther King Award for Achievement in Science and was recognized as one of the outstanding women in 100 years at the University of Connecticut. She was the winner of the Connecticut Technology Council Women of Innovation and Leadership Award and was recently elected Chair of the 2018 international Fibroblast Growth Factors in Development and Disease Gordon Conference. Dr. Hurley has also served as a permanent member of several NIH study section review panels.

Dr. Hurley is the Associate Dean for the Health Career Opportunity Programs and Founding Director of the Aetna Health Professions Partnership Initiative at UConn Health. This initiative, which began in 1996 as one of the 10 original medical school programs funded by the Robert Wood Johnson Foundation in response to the AAMC Project 3000 by 2000, is a consortium of several Connecticut partner colleges/universities and an urban school system designed to increase the awareness and preparedness of students from groups traditionally underepresented in the health professions.

At the local level, Dr. Hurley has presented to the Connecticut legislature and the Governor's Office for Workforce Development on the UConn Health Professions Partnership Initiative as a successful model of Connecticut Career Choices. In 2007, she was appointed to the Connecticut State Department of Education and the Department of Higher Education College Ready Advisory Subcommittee of the Higher Education PK-16 Council. In recognition of her contributions to educational diversity, Dr. Hurley has received numerous awards including the first New England Board of Higher Education Award for innovation and excellence in higher education; the West Indian Foundation Community Service Award; the Community Service Award from the Capital Area Health Consortium; and the Distinguished Service Award from the Foundation for Educational Achievement at Central Connecticut State University. She was also appointed Commissioner and served on the Connecticut Legislative Commission on Health Equity.

At the National level, Dr. Hurley served as Chair of the Women's Affairs Committee of the American Dental Education Association and was an invited speaker/panelist at The Sullivan Alliance National Leadership Symposium on Health Professions Diversity. Dr. Hurley was recently appointed to the Oversight Committee of NIH, NIDDK Network of Minority Health Research Investigators, and serves as UConn School of Medicine liaison to the AAMC Group on Women in Medicine and Science.

Camara Phyllis Jones, M.D., M.P.H., Ph.D., is Senior Fellow at the Satcher Health Leadership Institute and Cardiovascular Research Institute and Adjunct Associate Professor in the Department of Community Health and Preventive Medicine at the Morehouse School of Medicine. Previously, she was research director on social determinants of health and equity in the Division of Adult and Community Health, National Center for Chronic Disease Prevention and Health Promotion, Centers for Disease Control and Prevention. Dr. Jones received her B.A. degree (molecular biology) from Wellesley College, her M.D. from the Stanford University School of Medicine, and both her M.P.H. and Ph.D. (epidemiology) degrees from the Johns Hopkins School of Hygiene and Public Health. She also completed residency training in general preventive medicine (Johns Hopkins School of Hygiene and Public Health, Baltimore, Maryland) and in family practice (Residency Program in Social Medicine, Bronx, New York).

Dr. Jones is a family physician and epidemiologist whose work focuses on the impact of racism on the health and well-being of the nation. She seeks to broaden the national health debate to include not only universal access to high-quality health care but also attention to the social determinants of health (including poverty) and the social determinants of equity (including racism). As a methodologist, she has developed new ways for comparing full distributions of data (rather than means or proportions) in order to investigate population-level risk factors and propose population-level interventions. As a social epidemiologist, her work on race-associated differences in health outcomes goes beyond documenting those differences to vigorously investigating the structural causes of the differences. As a teacher, her allegories on race and racism illuminate topics that are otherwise difficult for many Americans to understand or discuss.

Darrell G. Kirch, M.D., is President and Chief Executive Officer of the AAMC. A distinguished physician, educator, and medical scientist, Dr. Kirch speaks and publishes widely on the need for transformation in the nation's health care system and how academic medicine can lead change across medical education, biomedical research, and patient care. His career spans all aspects of academic medicine and includes leadership positions at two medical schools and academic health systems, as well as at the NIH.

Before becoming AAMC president, Dr. Kirch was selected as chair-elect of the association, and cochaired the Liaison Committee on Medical Education, the accreditation body for medical schools. He also has served as chair of the AAMC Council of Deans Administrative Board and chair of the American Medical Association Section on Medical Schools.

Dr. Kirch assumed the position of AAMC president in July 2006 following 6 years as Senior Vice President for Health Affairs, dean of the college of medicine, and Chief Executive Officer of the Milton S. Hershey Medical Center at The Pennsylvania State University, where he and his leadership team are credited with revitalizing the institution and guiding it through a period of educational innovation and major growth in clinical activity and research funding. Before joining Penn State, Dr. Kirch held a number of leadership positions at the Medical College of Georgia from 1994 to 2000, including serving as dean of the medical school, senior vice president for clinical activities, and dean of the school of graduate studies.

As a psychiatrist and neuroscientist, Dr. Kirch conducted research on the biological basis of and clinical treatments for severe neuropsychiatric disorders. Following the completion of his residency training at the University of Colorado Health Sciences Center, he joined the National Institute of Mental Health (NIMH) in Bethesda, Maryland, where he was named acting scientific director in 1993. His NIMH contributions were recognized when he was presented with the Outstanding Service Medal of the U.S. Public Health Service.

Dr. Kirch is a member of several professional societies, including the American Psychiatric Association, American College of Psychiatrists, and American Medical Association, and he currently serves as chair of the Washington Higher Education Secretariat. He was elected to the National Academy of Medicine in 2007. In 2014, he was named a Distinguished Life Fellow by the American Psychiatric Association.

Michael G. Knight, M.D., MSHP, is an Assistant Professor of Medicine and Patient Safety Officer for the Division of General Internal Medicine of the GW Medical Faculty Associates. Dr. Knight completed undergraduate studies at Oakwood University, and obtained his Medical Degree with Special Qualifications in Biomedical Research from the Cleveland Clinic Lerner College of Medicine of Case Western Reserve University. During medical school, he participated in the year-long Clinical Research Training Program at the NIH, where his research focused on metabolic disease and obesity in women of African descent. He then completed residency in internal medicine, with special training in obesity medicine, at New York Presbyterian–Weill Cornell Medical Center.

He continued his training at the University of Pennsylvania as a Robert Wood Johnson Foundation Clinical Scholar and Fellow of the Leonard Davis Institute of Health Economics. While there, he completed a master's in health policy research, received training in LEAN Six Sigma, and led quality improvement and patient safety efforts in patient and provider communication, adverse event review, and transitions of care. He continued his training as a visiting fellow at The Joint Commission, where he focused on culture of safety development and sentinel event review.

While at the University of Pennsylvania, Dr. Knight also practiced clinically as an attending in internal medicine at the Crescenz VA Medical Center, and served as the clinical director for the MOVE! Level 3 Weight Management Program. In this role, he led a multidisciplinary team to provide medical weight management through nutrition, physical activity, and medication management. He also practiced clinically in general internal medicine, and focused on preventive medicine, chronic disease management, and coordination of care. Dr. Knight is board certified in internal medicine, and practices clinically with a focus in obesity medicine in the GW Weight Management Clinic and General Internal Medicine Practice.

Walter J. Lanier, J.D., is the Director of Multicultural Affairs and Community Engagement at Milwaukee Area Technical College (MATC), a multicampus community college with approximately 38,000 students. In 2015, Mr. Lanier led the design and launch of the college's Men of Color Initiative, which is designed to increase course completion, retention, and graduation rates of the college's men of color. Men of color are more than 22 percent of MATC's population; Black men are 56 percent of that total.

In addition to his work at MATC, Mr. Lanier is in his sixth year as the senior pastor of the Progressive Baptist Church of Milwaukee, Wisconsin. Progressive is very active in the Milwaukee community and is particularly recognized for its work in the areas of mental health, antiviolence, and HIV/AIDS prevention. In 2012, he formed "MIRACLE" (Mental Illness—Raising Awareness with Church and Community Leaders Everywhere), a collaboration of faith-based leaders, community leaders, and people with lived experience.

A 1995 graduate of the University of Michigan law school, Mr. Lanier maintained his own business law practice for over a decade prior to joining MATC. Mr. Lanier also lectured in the University of Wisconsin–Milwaukee Department of Africology in the areas of race and constitutional law.

He has served on numerous boards and is deeply committed to being a part of Milwaukee reaching its fullest potential. Mr. Lanier currently serves on a variety of community-wide boards including the Milwaukee County Mental Health Board, Milwaukee Community Justice Council, Milwaukee Inner City Congregations Allied for Hope, and Milwaukee Health Services, Inc.

Cato T. Laurencin, M.D., Ph.D., is a designated University Professor at the University of Connecticut (UConn). He is the Albert and Wilda Van Dusen Distinguished Endowed Chair Professor of Orthopaedic Surgery in the School of Medicine. In addition, Dr. Laurencin is a tenured member of the faculty in the School of Engineering and is Professor of Chemical and Biomolecular Engineering, Professor of Materials Engineering, and Professor of Biomedical Engineering at UConn. Dr. Laurencin serves as Chief Executive Officer of the Connecticut Institute for Clinical and Translational Science, UConn's cross-university translational science institute. In addition, he is the Founding Director of the Institute for Regenerative Engineering and the Founding Director of The Raymond and Beverly Sackler Center for Biomedical, Biological, Physical, and Engineering Sciences at UConn Health.

Dr. Laurencin is an elected member of the National Academy of Medicine and an elected member of the National Academy of Engineering.

Dr. Laurencin previously served as the UConn Health Center's Vice President for Health Affairs and Dean of the UConn School of Medicine. Prior to that Dr. Laurencin was the Lillian T. Pratt Distinguished Professor and Chair of the Department of Orthopedic Surgery at the University of Virginia, as well as the Orthopedic Surgeon-in-Chief at the University of Virginia Health System. In addition, he was designated as a University Professor at the University of Virginia by the President and held professorships in biomedical engineering and chemical engineering.

Dr. Laurencin earned his undergraduate degree in chemical engineering from Princeton University and his medical degree, magna cum laude, from the Harvard Medical School. During medical school, he also earned his Ph.D. in biochemical engineering/biotechnology from the Massachusetts Institute of Technology.

An expert in shoulder and knee surgery, Dr. Laurencin has been named to America's Top Doctors, and America's Top Surgeons. He is a Fellow of the American College of Surgeons, a Fellow of the American Academy of Orthopedic Surgeons, and is one of few orthopedic surgeons elected to the American Surgical Association. He is the winner of the Nicolas Andry Award from the Association of Bone and Joint Surgeons.

Dr. Laurencin's research involves tissue engineering, biomaterials science, nanotechnology and stem cell science, and a new field he terms *regenerative engineering*. He is an International Fellow in Biomaterials Science and Engineering and a Fellow of the American Institute for Medical and Biological Engineering, and a Fellow of the Biomedical Engineering Society. His work was honored by *Scientific American Magazine* as one of the 50 greatest achievements in science in 2007. Dr. Laurencin was named the 2009 winner of the Pierre Galletti Award, Medical and Institute of Chemical Engineers at its centennial celebration. Dr. Laurencin is active in technology development. In 2012 his work in musculoskeletal tissue regeneration was featured in *National Geographic Magazine*'s "100 Discoveries that Changed Our World" edition. In addition, he received the Technology, Innovation, and Development Award from the Society for Biomaterials in 2013 for key scientific and technical innovation and leadership in translational research.

Dr. Laurencin's work in mentoring students is well known. He received the Presidential Award for Excellence in Science, Mathematics, and Engineering Mentoring in ceremonies at the White House in 2010 and the Beckman Award for Mentoring in 2012. Most recently Dr. Laurencin was honored by the AAAS, receiving the AAAS Mentor Award.

Dr. Laurencin has lectured throughout the world on clinical orthopedic surgery and musculoskeletal research. He is an elected member of the Third World Academy of Sciences, and an elected member of the African Academy of Sciences.

Dr. Laurencin is active in science and health policy. He has been a member of the National Science Foundation's Advisory Committee for Engineering and has served both on the National Science Board of the Food and Drug Administration (FDA), and the National Advisory Council for Arthritis, Musculoskeletal, and Skin Diseases at the NIH. Dr. Laurencin is currently a member of the National Academies' Board on Life Sciences, and the National Academies' Division on Engineering and Physical Sciences. He currently holds appointments by the Secretary of Health and Human Services to the National Advisory Council for Biomedical Imaging and Bioengineering, and the Advisory Committee to the Director of the NIH.

John Lumpkin, M.D., M.P.H., is senior vice president for programs at the Robert Wood Johnson Foundation, where he is responsible for the Foundation's efforts aimed at transforming health and health care systems, ensuring that everyone has access to stable and affordable health care coverage, building leadership, and engaging business toward building a culture of health in the United States. These efforts help to catalyze fundamental changes in health and health care systems to achieve measurably better outcomes for all by maintaining high-quality, effective, and value-laden health care, public health, and population health services. Before joining the Foundation in April 2003, Dr. Lumpkin served as director of the Illinois Department of Public Health for 12 years. During his more than 17 years with the department, he served as acting director and prior to that as associate director.

Dr. Lumpkin has participated directly in the health and health care system, first practicing emergency medicine and teaching medical students and residents at The University of Chicago and Northwestern University. He is the past chairman of the board of directors of the Robert Wood Johnson University Hospital, the major teaching hospital of Rutgers University in New Brunswick. After earning his M.P.H. in 1985, he began caring for the more than 12 million people of Illinois as the first African American director of the state public health agency with more than 1,300 employees in seven regional offices, three laboratories, and locations in Springfield and Chicago. He led improvements to programs dealing with women's and men's health, information and technology, emergency and bioterrorism preparedness, infectious disease prevention and control, immunization, local health department coverage, and the state's laboratory services.

Dr. Lumpkin is a member of the National Academy of Medicine and a fellow of the American Academy of Nursing, American College of Emergency Physicians, and American College of Medical Informatics. He has been chairman of the National Committee on Vital and Health Statistics, and served on the U.S. Department of Agriculture's Council on Maternal, Infant, and Fetal Nutrition; the advisory committee to the director of the U.S. Centers for Disease Control and Prevention; and the Institute of Medicine's Committee on Assuring the Health of the Public in the 21st Century. He has served on the boards of directors for the Public Health Foundation and National Quality Forum, as president of the Illinois College of Emergency Physicians and the Society of Teachers of Emergency Medicine, and as speaker and board of directors' member of the American College of Emergency Physicians. He has received the Arthur McCormack Excellence and Dedication in Public Health Award from the Association of State and Territorial Health Officials, the Jonas Salk Health Leadership Award, and the Leadership in Public Health Award from the Illinois Public Health Association. Dr. Lumpkin also has been the recipient of the Bill B. Smiley Award, Alan Donaldson Award, African American History Maker, and Public Health Worker of the Year of the Illinois Public Health Association. He is the author of numerous journal articles and book chapters.

Dr. Lumpkin earned his M.D. and B.M.S. degrees from Northwestern University Medical School and his M.P.H. from the University of Illinois School of Public Health. He was the first African American trained in emergency medicine in the country after completing his residency at The

University of Chicago. He has served on the faculty of The University of Chicago, Northwestern University, and University of Illinois at Chicago.

Veronica T. Mallett, M.D., M.M.M., is Senior Vice President for Health Affairs and Dean of the School of Medicine at Meharry Medical College. In her role as Senior Vice President for Health Affairs, Dr. Mallett is responsible for the quality of health care provided at Meharry and for the maintenance of the health service affiliations that help the College provide exemplary training for its students, residents, and fellows.

As Dean of the School of Medicine, she serves as the chief academic and administrative officer of the medical school and oversees its academic programs, research efforts, curriculum, student affairs, and fiscal management. Dr. Mallett is also responsible for the academic component of residency programs.

Dr. Mallett has been recognized nationally and internationally for her work in the treatment of urinary incontinence and genital organ prolapse as well as her efforts to reduce health disparities. She joined Meharry from the Paul L. Foster School of Medicine at Texas Tech University Health Sciences Center El Paso where she served as founding chair and professor since March 2011. Prior to this position, she held faculty positions at Northwestern University, Wayne State University, and the University of Tennessee Health Science Center, serving in roles including Urogynecology Fellowship Director, Residency Director, Director of Health Care Excellence and Safety, Practice Plan Director, and Department Chair.

In addition to her impressive work as a researcher and educator, Dr. Mallett has made amazing strides in bettering health for people of Hispanic origin. Fluent in medical Spanish, she recently worked to develop a new medical school and health science center on the Texas/Mexico border aimed at addressing the critical physician shortage in El Paso and the surrounding community.

Dr. Mallett obtained her bachelor's degree in biology from Barnard University and received her M.D. from Michigan State University's College of Human Medicine. She also holds a master's degree in medical management from Carnegie Mellon University. She is board certified in obstetrics and gynecology, and female pelvic medicine and reconstructive pelvic surgery, and has authored nearly 100 articles, book chapters, and abstracts.

Alfred M. Mays, M.S., is a program officer at the Burroughs Wellcome Fund. Mr. Mays is responsible for managing grant competitions in science education and diversity of science. He also works closely with the North Carolina (NC) Science, Mathematics, and Technology Education Center. Prior to Alfred assuming this role, he served as an independent consultant with a service delivery that included strategic planning, project incubation, design, and implementation of a number initiatives within education agencies and organizations. Mr. Mays was the founder of EdSync Strategies, Inc., an education contract service that provided assistance to NC eLearning Commission, NC STEM (science, technology, engineering, and mathematics) Learning Network, rural NC public school systems, and the Public School Forum. From 2007 to 2011, he served as the assistant director of the Collaborative Project, an initiative that "sought to strengthen participating school systems serving low-income students in rural areas of the state." Mr. Mays has also worked with the University of North Carolina General Administration, serving as the director of information resources and director of special projects. Mr. Mays received his B.S. from Wilmington College and M.S. in administration from Central Michigan University. He served in the U.S. Air Force from 1984 to 1994, providing information system and data management support for various Air Force missions.

J. Michael McGinnis, M.D., M.P.P., a physician and epidemiologist, serves at the National Academy of Medicine (NAM) as Senior Scholar, Leonard D. Schaeffer Executive Officer, Executive Director of the Leadership Consortium for a Value & Science-Driven Health System and the NAM Learning Health System Initiative. He is also an elected member of the NAM (1999). Previously, Dr. McGinnis was Senior Vice President and head of the Health Group at the Robert Wood Johnson Foundation (1999–2005). Before that, he served as Assistant Surgeon General and Deputy Assistant Secretary for Health at the U.S. Department of Health and Human Services, with continuous leadership responsibility from 1977 to 1995 for federal activities in disease prevention and health promotion, a tenure unusual for political and policy posts. Chair and founder of various national efforts, key programs developed and launched at his initiative include the Healthy People national goals and objectives, the *Dietary Guidelines for Americans*, and the U.S. Preventive Services Task Force, each still ongoing. Internationally, he worked in India as state director for the WHO smallpox eradication program (1974–1975), and in Bosnia as Chair of the World Bank/European Commission Task Force for reconstruction in health and human services (1995–1996). Dr. McGinnis's scientific interests focus on population health and the determinants of health, his publications include approximately 200 articles and more than 20 edited books, and among his national recognitions are the public health Distinguished Service Medal (1989), Health Leader of the Year Award (1996), and Public Health Hero Award (2013). His degrees are from Berkeley (1966), UCLA (1971), and Harvard (1977); he was commencement speaker at each.

Roger A. Mitchell, Jr., M.D., is the Chief Medical Examiner for the Distirct of Columbia. Dr. Mitchell is board certified in anatomic and forensic pathology by the American Board of Pathology. He is a Fellow with the American Society of Clinical Pathology (FASCP) and the National Association of Medical Examiners (NAME). Dr. Mitchell sits on national subcommittees for NAME including Education & Planning and Strategic Planning.

He is a graduate of Howard University and UMDNJ-New Jersey Medical School. Dr. Mitchell is licensed to practice medicine in New Jersey and Washington, DC. He has performed more than 1,300 autopsy examinations in his career and has testified as an expert on numerous cases. He began the study of forensic science and violence prevention as a Forensic Biologist for the Federal Bureau of Investigation (FBI)–DNA Unit in January 1997 at the FBI Headquarters Building.

Dr. Mitchell served 4 years as the Assistant Deputy Chief Medical Examiner, in charge of Medicolegal Death Investigations, at the Harris County Institute of Forensic Sciences prior to serving 2 years as the Regional Medical Examiner for the Northern Regional Medical Examiner Office in Newark, New Jersey. Dr. Mitchell has served in large cities such as New York City, Houston, and Newark.

Dr. Mitchell has great interest in violence as a public health issue. He believes the medical examiner serves a critical role in public health prevention initiatives and continues to be at the forefront of issues relating to elder abuse and neglect and youth violence. He is recently published for his work on "Forensic Markers Associated with a History of Elder Mistreatment and Self Neglect" in the *Academic Forensic Pathology* journal.

Valerie Montgomery Rice, M.D., provides a valuable combination of experience at the highest levels of patient care and medical research, as well as organizational management and public health policy. Marrying her management skills and strategic thinking to tackle challenging problems, she has a track record of redesigning complex organizations' management infrastructures to reflect the needs of evolving strategic environments and position the organization for success.

The sixth president of Morehouse School of Medicine (MSM) and the first woman to lead the free-standing medical institution, Dr. Montgomery Rice serves as both the president and dean. A renowned infertility specialist and researcher, she most recently served as dean and executive vice president of MSM, where she served since 2011.

Prior to joining MSM, Dr. Montgomery Rice held faculty positions and leadership roles at various health centers, including academic health centers. Most notably, she was the founding director of the Center for Women's Health Research at Meharry Medical College, one of the nation's first research centers devoted to studying diseases that disproportionately impact women of color.

Dedicated to the creation and advancement of health equity, Dr. Montgomery Rice lends her vast experience and talents to programs that enhance pipeline opportunities for academically diverse students, diversifies the physician and scientific workforce, and fosters equity in health care access and health outcomes. To this end she holds membership in many organizations and boards, such as the National Academy of Medicine (2016–present), National Center for Advancing Translational Sciences (2016–present), Board of Directors for Kaiser Permanente School of Medicine (2016–present), Board of Directors for the Nemours Foundation (2016–present), The Josiah Macy Jr. Foundation (2017–present), and the Association of American Medical Colleges Council of Deans.

Dr. Montgomery Rice has received numerous accolades and honors. She was named to the Horatio Alger Association of Distinguished Americans and a recipient of the 2017 Horatio Alger Award. For 2 consecutive years (2016, 2017) *Georgia Trend Magazine* selected Dr. Montgomery Rice as one of the 100 Most Influential Georgians. Other honors include the Trumpet Vanguard Award (2015); the Dorothy Heights Crystal Stair Award (2014); National Coalition of 100 Black Women–Women of Impact (2014); YWCA–Women of Achievement (Atlanta in 2014 and Nashville in 2007); American Medical Women's Association Elizabeth Blackwell Medal (2011); and Working Mother Media Multicultural Women's Legacy Award (2011).

A Georgia native, Dr. Montgomery Rice holds a bachelor's degree in chemistry from the Georgia Institute of Technology and a medical degree from Harvard Medical School. She completed her residency in obstetrics and gynecology at Emory University School of Medicine and her fellowship in reproductive endocrinology and infertility at Hutzel Hospital in Detroit, Michigan.

Randall C. Morgan, Jr., M.D., M.B.A., is the Executive Director of the W. Montague Cobb/NMA Health Institute and an orthopedic surgeon who practices in Sarasota and Bradenton, Florida. After serving as founder and President of University Park Orthopedics in that community, he has become a partner in the Sarasota Orthopedic Associates. Dr. Morgan served as the 95th President of the National Medical Association during the years 1996 and 1997. He was the first board-certified orthopedic surgeon to hold that position. Dr. Morgan is a true pioneer in his profession and was among the first surgeons to perform total joint replacement surgery at Northwestern University.

Dr. Morgan has practiced medicine in Evanston, Illinois, and well as in his hometown of Gary, Indiana, for more than 30 years prior to his relocation to Sarasota. With the assistance of his father, Mr. Randall C. Morgan, Sr., he founded the Orthopedic Centers of Northwest Indiana and served as its president from 1975 to 1999. At one time, this was the largest minority-owned orthopedic practice in the United States. He is a Diplomat of the American Board of Orthopedic Surgery and the American Board of Managed Care Medicine. He is also a Fellow of the American College of Surgeons.

James L. Moore III, Ph.D., is the Interim Vice Provost for Diversity and Inclusion and Chief Diversity Officer at The Ohio State University, where he is also the College of Education and Human Ecology Distinguished Professor of Urban Education in the College of Education and Human Ecology and inaugural executive director of the Todd Anthony Bell National Resource Center on the African American Male. From 2011 to 2015, he was an associate provost for Diversity and Inclusion, where he managed numerous programs and units, including the Morrill Scholarship Program, Office of Diversity and Inclusion Scholars Program, Young Scholars Program, Upward Bound of Columbus, Upward Bound of Wooster, Community Outreach, Todd Anthony Bell National Resource Center on the African American Male, and Administration/ Special Programs.

Dr. Moore received his B.A. in English education from Delaware State University and earned both his M.A.Ed. and Ph.D. in counselor education from Virginia Polytechnic Institute and State University (a.k.a., Virginia Tech). As a scholar, he has a national- and international-recognized research agenda that focuses on the following: (a) how educational professionals, such as school counselors, influence the educational/career aspirations and school experiences of students of color (particularly African American males); (b) sociocultural, familial, school, and community factors that support, enhance, and impede academic outcomes for preK–12 African American students (e.g., elementary, secondary, and postsecondary); (c) recruitment and retention issues of students of color, particularly African Americans, in preK–12 gifted education and those high-potential college students in STEM majors; and (d) social, emotional, and psychological consequences of racial oppression for African American males and other people of color in various domains in society (e.g., education, counseling, workplace, athletics).

Since beginning his professional career as an academic, Dr. Moore has made significant contributions to the fields of school counseling, gifted education, urban education, multicultural counseling/education, higher education, and STEM education. More specifically, he has published over 100 refereed articles, editor-reviewed articles, book chapters, special theme issues, and so on.

Marc A. Nivet, Ed.D., M.B.A., is the Executive Vice President for Institutional Advancement at UT Southwestern Medical Center, where he provides strategic vision and oversight in coordinating the areas of development; communications, marketing, and public affairs; government affairs; and community and corporate relations. Prior to his role at UT Southwestern, Dr. Nivet served as a member of the executive leadership team of the AAMC, where he provided leadership on issues surrounding community engagement, diversity, and health equity at medical schools and teaching hospitals across the United States and Canada.

Prior to his position at the AAMC, Dr. Nivet served from 2005 to 2010 as the Chief Operating Officer and Treasurer of The Josiah Macy Jr. Foundation in New York, a national foundation focused on the education of health professionals. He concurrently served from 2008 to 2010 as Special Assistant to the Senior Vice President of Health at New York University, and held earlier positions involved in program planning and evaluation, financial management, grant development and review, media relations, and issues of access and diversity in medical school admissions.

Dr. Nivet earned his doctoral degree in higher education management from the University of Pennsylvania and an M.B.A. with a focus on health care management from The George Washington University's School of Business. He has a bachelor of science degree in communication studies from Southern Connecticut State University. He is a fellow of The New York Academy of Medicine, and a former President of the National Association of Medical Minority Educators.

Elizabeth Ofili, M.D., is Professor of Medicine and Director and Senior Associate Dean, Clinical Research Center and Clinical and Translational Research, at the Morehouse School of Medicine. She is a national and internationally recognized clinician scientist with particular focus on cardiovascular disparities and women's health. Dr. Ofili has been continuously funded by the NIH and industry/foundations since 1994, with a track record in clinical trials that impact health disparities. In 2002, as president of the Association of Black Cardiologists, she led the initiative to implement the landmark African American Heart Failure Trial, whose findings led to a change in practice guidelines for the treatment of heart failure in African Americans.

Over the past 17 years, she has led the growth of the clinical research infrastructure and training programs at Morehouse School of Medicine with awards totaling more than $150 million, including serving as the founding director of the U54 center of clinical research excellence, the community physicians network, the U54 Research Centers in Minority Institutions (RCMI) Center of Excellence for Clinical and Translational Research, and the R25 clinical research education and career development program. Dr. Ofili has mentored more than 30 M.D. and Ph.D. clinical and translational science investigators, many of whom remain at MSM. She has mentored more than 25 underrepresented minority STEM undergraduates and high school students through funding from NASA and the Minority Biomedical Research Students program.

She is the senior co-PI of the Atlanta Clinical and Translational Science Institute (ACTSI), a citywide collaborative Clinical and Translational Science Awards program at Emory University, Morehouse School of Medicine, and Georgia Institute of Technology, along with their partnering health systems and statewide research organizations. Since 2007, ACTSI has engaged more than 673 investigators, and 134 postdoctoral and predoctoral trainees in discovery science, training, and community engagement. Dr. Ofili has led successful multi-institutional collaborations through the ACTSI and the RCMI Translational Research Network of 18 historically Black, Hispanic, and Minority Serving Institutions (MSIs) across the nation, and was lead author of a publication on models of partnerships between HBCUs/MSIs and research intensive institutions.

Dr. Ofili holds a patent for "A system and method for chronic illness care," and is the recipient of more than 20 national and international awards, including the 2003 National Library of Medicine's "Changing the Face of Medicine, the Rise of America's Women," the Daniel Savage Memorial Science Award from the Association of Black Cardiologists, America's Top Doctors by *Black Enterprise Magazine,* and 100 Most influential health care leaders by *Atlanta Business Chronicle.*

She has delivered more than 600 scientific presentations and published more than 130 scientific papers in national and international journals. As an AAMC 2007 Council of Dean Fellow, Dr. Ofili led a project on best practices to sustaining the biomedical and physician workforce. She has advised the NIH on diversity in the biomedical research workforce, and currently serves on the Advisory Board of the National Clinical Center (NIH), and on the AAMC advisory panel on research. She is an elected member of the Association of University Cardiologists, and is on the board of directors of the National Space Biomedical Research Institute.

William F. Owen, Jr., M.D., FACP, is Dean and Chancellor of Ross University School of Medicine (Ross). He is an accomplished medical academician, experienced clinician, highly respected scientific researcher, and a leader in global health sciences education. Immediately prior to joining Ross, Dr. Owen was the Dean of Medical Sciences at American University of the Caribbean School of Medicine (AUC), a sister medical school within Adtalem Global Education.

A native of Memphis, Tennessee, Dr. Owen is a graduate of Phillips Academy and Brown University. He earned his M.D. with high honors from Tufts University School of Medicine in 1980, and trained in internal medicine and nephrology at Harvard Medical School's Brigham and Women's Hospital, where he was a Robert Wood Johnson Foundation Fellow in the Minority Medical Faculty Development Program. At Harvard he was a full-time faculty member, and later went on to serve as a tenured professor at three institutions—Duke University, the University of Tennessee, and AUC. He was a Visiting Professor at Imperial College London in its Institute of Global Health Innovation, and at the National University of Singapore.

In a stellar career that has included many firsts, Dr. Owen served as the first African American Chancellor and Senior Vice President of Health Affairs at the University of Tennessee, where he led the College of Medicine and five other health professions colleges. He then served for 5 years as President of the University of Medicine and Dentistry of New Jersey, the statewide health education and medical services component of Rutgers University, the largest publicly funded academic health system in the United States. In this role Dr. Owen was responsible for two allopathic medical schools and an osteopathic medical school, as well as colleges of nursing, public health, allied health, dentistry, graduate medical sciences, and several large magnet teaching hospitals and research institutes.

In 2012 he was appointed the inaugural Chief Executive Officer of Sidra Medical and Research Center in Qatar, the major international training site for Weill Cornell Medical College. He was also the inaugural health policy advisor to the President of the International Association of University Presidents, a nongovernmental organization that advises the United Nations on matters of higher education.

The recipient of numerous accolades and awards, Dr. Owen has been honored in the *Congressional Record*, featured in *Ebony Magazine*, and listed in several *Who's Who* publications, among others. He has received approximately $10 million in biomedical research grants and has more than 180 peer-reviewed articles, chapters, and books to his credit. In 2006 Dr. Owen was an inventor on a federal patent issued for "Methods and compositions for detection of microbial contaminants in peritoneal dialysis solutions."

Luis Padilla, M.D., FAAFP, is the Associate Administrator for Health Workforce at the Health Resources and Services Administration (HRSA). He also serves as director of the National Health Service Corps (NHSC). HRSA is an agency of the U.S. Department of Health and Human Services (HHS). Prior to joining the Bureau of Health Workforce at HRSA, Dr. Padilla was senior health policy advisor to the Chief Executive Officer of Unity Health Care in Washington, DC, a federally qualified health center network with more than 100,000 patients. He also served as Unity's research director and sought academic partnerships with an emphasis on community-based participatory research. A committed advocate for the underserved, Dr. Padilla is a former NHSC Scholar who completed his service at Upper Cardozo Health Center, where he became the medical director. He was also appointed to the National Advisory Council of the NHSC from 2007 to 2010. A board-certified family physician, Dr. Padilla received a B.A. in philosophy and a B.S. in biology from the University of California, Irvine. He earned his medical degree from Wake Forest School of Medicine and completed his family medicine residency at Brown University.

Vivian Pinn, M.D., was the first full-time Director of the NIH Office of Research on Women's Health, an appointment she held since 1991 and as NIH Associate Director for Research on Women's Health since 1994 prior to her retirement in August 2011. Since her retirement, she has been named as a Senior Scientist Emerita at the NIH Fogarty International Center. Dr. Pinn came to NIH from Howard University College of Medicine in Washington, DC, where she had been Professor and Chair of the Department of Pathology from 1982 until 1991. Dr. Pinn had previously held teaching appointments at Harvard Medical School and Tufts University where she was also Assistant Dean for Student Affairs. A special tribute by Senator Olympia Snowe on Dr. Pinn's retirement was published in the *Congressional Record* in November 2011 commending her contributions during her NIH tenure. The Association of American Medical Colleges awarded her a Special Recognition Award for exceptional leadership over a 40-year career.

She has received numerous honors and recognitions, and is a fellow of the American Academy of Arts and Sciences and was elected to the National Academy of Medicine in 1995. A graduate and Alumna Achievement Award recipient as well as former Trustee of Wellesley College, she earned her M.D. from the University of Virginia School of Medicine, the only woman or minority in her class. She completed her postgraduate training in pathology at the Massachusetts General Hospital. Dr. Pinn has received 14 honorary degrees of science, law, and medicine, and the University of Virginia School of Medicine has named one of its four advisory medical student colleges as "The Pinn College" in her honor. Tufts University School of Medicine in 2011 announced the "The Vivian W. Pinn Office of Student Affairs," named for her at the time her former medical students dedicated a scholarship in her name. She has held leadership positions in many professional organizations, including President of the National Medical Association (NMA), and is currently Chair of the NMA Past Presidents Council. Dr. Pinn currently serves on the Board of Trustees/Advisors of Thomas Jefferson University and Tufts University

School of Medicine. She was recently elected to Modern Healthcare's Hall of Fame, the first African American woman to be so honored, and received the Outstanding Woman Leader in Healthcare Award from the University of Michigan.

Wizdom Powell, Ph.D., is Director of the Health Disparities Institute and Associate Professor of Psychiatry at UConn Health. Formerly, Dr. Powell was Associate Professor of Health Behavior at the University of North Carolina (UNC) at Chapel Hill's Gillings School of Global Public Health, and Research Associate Professor in UNC's Department of Social Medicine. Dr. Powell also served as Associate Director of the Center for Health Equity Research, faculty member at UNC's Lineberger Comprehensive Cancer Center, and Director of the UNC's Men's Health Research Lab.

In 2011–2012, she was appointed by President Obama to serve as a White House Fellow to Secretary of Defense Leon Panetta. In this role she provided subject matter expertise on military mental health (e.g., posttraumatic stress disorder, suicide, and military sexual trauma). Her community-based research focuses on of the role of modern racism and gender norms on African American male health outcomes and health care inequities. She has published numerous peer-reviewed articles and book chapters, including ones in the *American Journal of Public Health, Journal of General Internal Medicine, Behavioral Medicine*, and *Child Development*.

In addition to being a White House Fellow, she is an American Psychological Association (APA) Minority, Robert Wood Johnson Foundation, Kaiser Permanente Burch, Institute of African American Research, and Ford Foundation Fellow who received a Ph.D. and an M.S. in clinical psychology and an M.P.H. from the University of Michigan, Ann Arbor. She serves as chair of the APA's workgroup on Health Disparities in Boys and Men and cochair of the Health Committee for President Obama's My Brother's Keeper Initiative in Durham County.

In recognition of her public service to boys and men, she received the American Psychological Association's (D51) Distinguished Professional Service Award. In 2015, she received the prestigious Phillip and Ruth Hettleman Prize for Outstanding Artistic and Scholarly Achievement by Young Faculty. Dr. Powell was awarded a 2017 academic writing residency at the Bellagio Center from the Rockefeller Foundation. During this highly competitive residency, Dr. Powell will work with other global leaders on strategies for transforming social and health care system landscapes to address gendered health inequities among vulnerable males. Most recently, she was selected as a Health Innovator Fellow by the Aspen Institute.

Deborah Prothrow-Stith, M.D., is Dean and Professor of Medicine for the College of Medicine at the Charles R. Drew University of Medicine and

Science in Los Angeles. Prior to her joing Drew University, Dr. Prothrow-Stith was a consultant at Spencer Stuart for executive searches for public health and health care services organizations and health professional associations. Previously, Dr. Prothrow-Stith served as associate dean and professor of public health practice at the Harvard School of Public Health. She is recognized as one of the creators of a nationwide social movement to prevent violence, and is the coauthor of several books: *Deadly Consequences*, the first book to present the public health perspective on the topic to a mass audience; *Sugar and Spice and No Longer Nice; Murder Is No Accident*; and *Health Skills for Wellness*, a state-of the-art high school health text.

As a board-certified internist, Dr. Prothrow-Stith has extensive clinical experience including service as attending physician at Boston City Hospital and chief of the Adolescent Clinic at Harvard Street Neighborhood Health Center. Appointed by the governor, Dr. Prothrow-Stith served as the Massachusetts public health commissioner with responsibility for seven hospitals, 3,500 employees, and a $350 million budget. In that role, she expanded treatment programs for AIDS patients, increased funding for drug rehabilitation, and launched a statewide office to prevent youth violence.

In addition to 10 honorary doctorates, Dr. Prothrow-Stith has received the 1993 World Health Day Award, the 1989 Secretary of Health and Human Service Award, and a presidential appointment to the National Commission on Crime Control and Prevention. In 2003, she was inducted to the National Academy of Medicine, one of academic medicine's highest achievements. Dr. Prothrow-Stith is a graduate of Spelman College and Harvard Medical School.

Sohi Rastegar, Ph.D.,[2] is a Senior Advisor and the Head of the Office of Emerging Frontiers and Multidisciplinary Activities at the U.S. National Science Foundation (NSF), Directorate for Engineering. He joined NSF in November 2003 following 15 years of academic and administrative service at Texas A&M University, Virginia Commonwealth University, and the Johns Hopkins University. He has been an Invited Professor at the Swiss Institute of Technology in Lausanne, Switzerland. He earned his B.S. (with highest honors) and M.S. in aerospace engineering, and his Ph.D. in biomedical engineering at The University of Texas at Austin. Dr. Rastegar has more than 150 scientific publications and presentations and has trained 8 Ph.D. and 14 M.S. students. He is a cofounder of BioTex, Inc., a medical device company in Houston, Texas. He is a Fellow of the American Institute for Medical and Biological Engineering, a Fellow of the American Society for Lasers in Medicine and Surgery, has served

[2] Sohi Rastegar was unable to attend the meeting.

as the Chair of Bioengineering Division of American Society of Mechanical Engineers, Associate Editor of *Annals of Biomedical Engineering*, and a member of the editorial boards of the *Journal of Biomedical Optics* and *Journal of Diabetes Science and Technology*. Dr. Rastegar is the recipient of awards and honors including the Select Young Faculty Award from the Texas Engineering Experiment Station, and the Director's Superior Accomplishment Award from the National Science Foundation.

Joan Y. Reede, M.D., M.S., M.P.H., M.B.A., is the first Dean for Diversity and Community Partnership, responsible for the development and management of a comprehensive program that provides leadership, guidance, and support to promote the increased recruitment, retention, and advancement of underrepresented minority faculty at Harvard Medical School (HMS). This charge includes oversight of all diversity activities at HMS as they relate to faculty, trainees, students, and staff.

In 1990, Dr. Reede founded the HMS Minority Faculty Development Program and also currently serves as Faculty Director of the Community Outreach programs. In 2008, she became the Director of the Harvard Catalyst Program for Faculty Development and Diversity. In addition, Dr. Reede holds appointments of Professor of Medicine at the Massachusetts General Hospital Institute for Health Policy and Associate Director of Leadership Development and Professor of Society and Behavioral Sciences at the Harvard T.H. Chan School of Public Health.

In 1989, prior to coming to HMS, Dr. Reede served as the medical director of a Boston community health center, and the Commonwealth of Massachusetts Department of Youth Services. She has also worked as a pediatrician in community and academic health centers, juvenile prisons, and public schools.

Dr. Reede created and developed more than 20 programs at HMS that aim to address pipeline and leadership issues for minorities and women who are interested in careers in medicine, academic and scientific research, and the health care professions. Supported by a dedicated staff, she has developed mentoring programs for underrepresented minority students from the middle school through the graduate and medical school levels. She has also designed a training program for middle and high school teachers, developed science curricula for public schools, implemented research and exchange clerkship programs at HMS, and designed and implemented innovative fellowships in minority health policy for physicians, dentists, and doctoral-level mental health professionals.

In collaboration with the Massachusetts Medical Society and the New England Board of Higher Education, Dr. Reede founded the Biomedical Science Careers Program (BSCP). A collaborative, community-based organization, BSCP's scope of involvement includes academia, private industry, medical centers, public education, and professional societies. BSCP's goal is to identify, support, and provide mentoring for underrepresented minority students, trainees, and professionals pursuing careers in the biomedical and health sciences. Dr. Reede has served on numerous advisory committees and panels at the state and national levels.

Dr. Reede graduated from Brown University and Mount Sinai School of Medicine. She completed a pediatric residency at Johns Hopkins Hospital in Baltimore, Maryland, and a fellowship in child psychiatry at Boston Children's Hospital. She holds an M.P.H. and an M.S. in health policy management from the Harvard T.H. Chan School of Public Health, and an M.B.A. from Boston University.

David Satcher, M.D., Ph.D.,[3] is a physician–scientist and public health administrator with an extensive track record of leadership, research, and community engagement. He is a Phi Beta Kappa graduate of Morehouse College and holds M.D. and Ph.D. degrees from Case Western Reserve University. Dr. Satcher served as the 16th Surgeon General of the United States (1998–2002) and the 10th Assistant Secretary for Health in the U.S. Department of Health and Human Services (1998–2001). He also served as Director of the Centers for Disease Control and Prevention and Administrator of the Agency for Toxic Substances and Disease Registry. Dr. Satcher has also held top leadership positions at the Charles R. Drew University for Medicine and Science, Meharry Medical College, and the Morehouse School of Medicine. He has received more than 50 honorary degrees and has received numerous awards from diverse organizations and agencies. Currently, Dr. Satcher is the Founding Director and Senior Advisor for the Satcher Health Leadership Institute at the Morehouse School of Medicine, Atlanta, Georgia.

Louis W. Sullivan, M.D., is the Chairman and Chief Executive Officer of The Sullivan Alliance to Transform the Health Professions. He is also chairman of the board of the National Health Museum in Atlanta, Georgia, which aims to improve the health of Americans by enhancing health literacy and advancing healthy behaviors. Dr. Sullivan served as chair of the President's Commission on Historically Black Colleges and Universities from 2002 to 2009 and was cochair of the President's Commission on HIV and AIDS from 2001 to 2006. With the exception of his tenure as secretary of the U.S. Department of Health and Human Services (HHS) from 1989 to 1993, Dr. Sullivan was president of Morehouse School of Medicine (MSM) for more than two decades.

---

[3] David Satcher was unable to attend the meeting.

As Secretary of HHS, Dr. Sullivan's efforts to improve the health and health behavior of Americans included (1) the introduction of a new and improved FDA food label; (2) release of *Healthy People 2000*, a guide for improved health promotion/disease prevention activities; (3) education of the public about health dangers from tobacco use; (4) successful efforts to prevent the introduction of "Uptown," a non-filtered, mentholated cigarette by R.J. Reynolds Tobacco Company; (5) inauguration of a $100 million minority male health and injury prevention initiative; and (6) implementation of greater gender and ethnic diversity in senior positions of HHS, including the appointment of the first female director of the NIH, the first female and first Hispanic Surgeon General of the U.S. Public Health Service, and the first African American Commissioner of the Social Security Administration.

Hannah Valantine, M.D., M.R.C.P., received her Bachelor of Medicine, Bachelor of Surgery (M.B.B.S.; the United Kingdom's equivalent to an M.D.) from St. George's Hospital, London University, in 1978. After that, she moved to the University of Hong Kong Medical School for specialty training in elective surgery before returning to the United Kingdom. She was awarded a diploma of membership by the Royal College of Physicians (M.R.C.P.) in 1981. In addition, she completed postgraduate training and numerous fellowships, serving as senior house officer in Cardiology at Brompton Hospital and Registrar in Cardiology and General Medicine at Hammersmith Hospital. In 1985, Dr. Valantine moved to the United States for postdoctoral training in cardiology at Stanford University, and in 1988, she received a Doctor of Science (D.Sc.), Medicine, from London University. Dr. Valantine became a Clinical Assistant Professor in the Cardiology Division at Stanford and rose through the academic ranks to become a full Professor of Medicine in the Division of Cardiovascular Medicine and Director of Heart Transplantation Research. She came to the NHLBI in 2014 to continue her research while also serving as the first NIH Chief Officer of Scientific Workforce Diversity. Dr. Valantine has received numerous awards throughout her career including a Best Doctor in America honor in 2002. She has authored more than 160 primary research articles and reviews and previously served on the editorial boards of the journals *Graft* and *Ethnicity & Disease*. Dr. Valantine is a member of the American College of Cardiology, the American Society of Transplant Physicians, and the American Heart Association, and past President of the American Heart Association Western States Affiliate.

C. Reynold Verret, Ph.D., is the sixth president of Xavier University of Louisiana and the University's second lay president. Prior to his appointment at Xavier, Dr. Verret served as provost and chief academic officer for Savannah State University. He served also as provost at Wilkes University in Pennsylvania and as Dean of the Misher College of Arts and Sciences and Professor of Chemistry and Biochemistry, University of the Sciences in Philadelphia. At these institutions, he led the revisions of general education curricula, oversaw accreditations, developed international programs, established collaborative agreements with neighboring institutions at the K–12 and higher education levels, instituted new state-approved academic programs, promoted interdisciplinary efforts between the humanities and sciences, and planned new facilities. Dr. Verret also served on faculty at Tulane University and also at Clark Atlanta University, where he was chair of the department of chemistry for many years.

As a scientist, Dr. Verret's research interests have included the cytotoxicity of immune cells, biosensors, and biomarkers. He has published in the fields of biological chemistry and immunology. At the University of the Sciences, he led a faculty effort establishing a knowledge network on social exclusion in support of the Commission on Social Determinants of Health within the World Health Organization.

Throughout, Dr. Verret has worked to enhance student achievement and progression to degree. He has contributed to increasing the number of U.S. students pursuing degrees in STEM disciplines and continuing to advanced study. This has included initiatives to mitigate the shortage of qualified science and math teachers in K–12.

He has served on many professional organizations and advisory bodies, including those of the NIH, the Board of the Pennsylvania Humanities Council, and the Georgia Coastal Indicators Coalition. He has received awards and fellowships for teaching and scholarship.

Dr. Verret received his undergraduate degree cum laude in biochemistry from Columbia University and the Ph.D. in biochemistry from the Massachusetts Institute of Technology (MIT). To these, were added postdoctoral experiences as fellow at the Howard Hughes Institute for Immunology at Yale and the Center for Cancer Research at MIT.

Adrienne White-Faines, M.P.A., FACHE, serves as Chief Executive Officer of the American Osteopathic Association (AOA), which represents more than 129,000 osteopathic physicians (DOs) and osteopathic medical students. Ms. White-Faines leads the AOA's strategic agenda, supporting the organization's physician and student members by promoting public health and advancing research; serving as the accrediting agency for osteopathic medical schools; and provider of physician specialty board certification and continuing medical education.

For 10 years prior to joining the AOA, Ms. White-Faines served as vice president of health initiatives and advocacy at the American Cancer Society, Illinois Division, where she was accountable for cancer research, education, advocacy, and patient service programs. Prior to employment at the American Cancer Society, she served as chief operating officer at Chicago-based Renwal Emergency Medical Services, a health care management consulting firm for hospitals and physicians, and at Chicago's Northwestern Memorial Hospital, where she oversaw a $600 million hospital redevelopment project. She also worked as a health strategist with the New York City Health and Hospitals Corporation, and as a practice administrator for a large physician group practice in Whittier, California.

Ms. White-Faines remains active with numerous Chicago and national nonprofit organizations, including the Erikson Institute, American Field Service-USA, and as a fellow with Leadership Greater Chicago. She holds a master of public administration from the University of Southern California in Los Angeles and a bachelor of arts from Amherst (Massachusetts) College.

M. Roy Wilson, M.D., is the 12th president of Wayne State University, where he has realigned the university's numerous research divisions to emphasize team science and cluster hiring of scientists. This effort was reflected in the organization of the science teams in the $90 million IBio multidisciplinary research facility, which opened in 2015. He also developed a strategy to improve the pipeline of underrepresented students toward science careers. As part of this strategy, he formed a coalition of Detroit-based universities and colleges to launch the NIH-funded Building Infrastructure Leading to Diversity Program at the university in 2015. In an effort to increase the diversity of Wayne State's campus, Dr. Wilson created the position of Associate Provost for Diversity and Inclusion and Chief Diversity Officer in 2014. He also created the Office of Multicultural Student Engagement to provide an inclusive environment and promote awareness initiatives that encourage academic success for underrepresented minorities and historically marginalized students.

Prior to joining Wayne State, Dr. Wilson served as deputy director for strategic scientific planning and program coordination at the National Institute on Minority Health and Health Disparities of the NIH. Previously, he was dean of the School of Medicine and vice president for health sciences at Creighton University, president of the Texas Tech University Health Sciences Center, and concurrently, chancellor of the University of Colorado Denver and chair of the Board of Directors of University of Colorado Hospital. Dr. Wilson also chaired the Board of Directors of the Charles R. Drew University of Medicine and Science and was acting president during part of that time.

Dr. Wilson's research has focused on glaucoma and blindness in populations from the Caribbean to West Africa. He was elected a lifetime member of the National Academy of Medicine in 2003. He received his undergraduate degree from Allegheny College, an M.S. in epidemiology from the University of California, Los Angeles, and an M.D. from Harvard Medical School.

Additional honors include the American Academy of Ophthalmology's Senior Achievement Award, the Distinguished Physician Award from the Minority Health Institute, the Herbert W. Nickens Award from the Association of American Medical Colleges, the NIH Director's Award, and the Cato T. Laurencin Distinguished Research Career Award from the National Medical Association. He received an honorary doctor of humane letters from Allegheny College in 2016.

STUDENTS PARTICIPATING IN WORKSHOP

Martin Campbell is a 2nd-year medical student at Morehouse School of Medicine. He attended Morehouse College, where he obtained a bachelor of science degree in biology. He served as the community service cochair for the 1st-year M.D. class and the community service chair for the Christian Medical and Dental Association at Morehouse School of Medicine. Mr. Campbell also served as the 1st-year liaison for the Internal Medicine Interest Group. In Mr. Campbell's 1st year of medical school, he cofounded Crossroads ministry, which is a student-led organization focused on tailoring to the spiritual growth and health of students through bible studies, community outreach, and fellowship events. This past summer, Mr. Campbell did an intensive 8-week research program at the Centers for Disease Control and Prevention (CDC) in Atlanta, Georgia. As part of his research project, he helped optimize a novel bead-based Luminex multiplex immunoassay for the detection of IgG antibodies against measles and rubella in rhesus macaques while simultaneously optimizing it for use in human serum. He presented his findings before CDC and program faculty, and his efforts have contributed to the global undertaking of eradicating measles and rubella infections worldwide. In addition, Mr. Campbell is an active member of the Student National Medical Association and American Society of Clinical Oncology.

Prior to entering medical school, Mr. Campbell lived in College Station, Texas, where he worked at the Texas A&M Veterinary Medical Diagnostic Lab (TVMDL) as an Analytical Chemistry Technician. During his 2 years in that role, he developed a method for simultaneously detecting three isomers of vitamin A and two isomers of vitamin E in animal serum and liver via high performance liquid chromatography. Mr. Campbell also developed a method to detect selenium levels in animal tissue using graphite furnace atomic absorption spectrometry and microwave-assisted tissue digestion. While working at TVMDL, Mr. Campbell also worked as a Clinical Laboratory Technician at Baylor Scott and White hospital, where he became proficient in phlebotomy, specimen processing, urinalysis, and ELISA testing.

Michael Denning is a current 2nd-year undergraduate student at East Carolina University. Currently, he is participating in a combined degree program, and will be graduating next year with a bachelor of science in public health studies and a master of business administration. In addition to being an EC Scholar and Early Assurance in Medicine Scholar to the Brody School of Medicine, he is active in several clubs and organizations on and off campus, all of which focus on promoting equity and equality for minorities, students, and rural community members, especially in the fields of health care, youth development, and educational attainment and preparation.

Gabriel Felix is a 3rd-year medical student at Howard University College of Medicine. He attended Binghamton University in New York, where he received his bachelor of arts in psychology. Prior to medical school he worked at the Kessler Foundation doing research on survivors of traumatic brain injuries and individuals living with disabilities. He currently serves as the National President-elect for the Student National Medical Association and sits as a trustee for the National Medical Association. He hopes to use his position to continue to support medical and premedical students to become culturally competent and socially conscious physicians that advocate for underserved communities.

Ross McMillan is an M.D./Ph.D. candidate at the Johns Hopkins University School of Medicine. He is from Tallahassee, Florida, and attended Morehouse College, where he earned a bachelor of science degree in biology. He then matriculated to Johns Hopkins University School of Medicine, where he joined the lab of Dr. William Matsui. His thesis focused on the characterization and therapeutic targeting of pancreatic cancer stem cells. While at Hopkins, he also served as the Regional Director for Region VI of the Student National Medical Association. He is currently applying for residency into the field of internal medicine and in the future hopes to work as a medical educator, translational researcher, and diversity practitioner.

Abbas Rattani, M.Be., is currently a 3rd-year medical student at Loyola University Chicago Stritch School of Medicine. This past year he served as a Paul Farmer Global Surgery Research Associate with the Program for Global Surgery and Social Change at Harvard Medical School and a Fellow with the Vanderbilt Medical Scholars Program at Vanderbilt University School of Medicine. He is also a founder and the current director of the creative arts nonprofit #MIPSTERZ, which has been featured on CNN, CBS, NPR, and *The Atlantic*. His research interests include neurological diseases, bioethics, Islamic studies, social justice, cost-effectiveness analysis, and health systems research in low- and middle-income countries. He is an alumnus of the University of North Carolina at Chapel Hill and the University of Pennsylvania.

Khalil Taylor is a graduate student in the Interdisciplinary Health Science program at Drexel University in Philadelphia, Pennsylvania. He received his B.S. from Villanova University in 2016 and double majored in biology and psychology. He is a Gates Millennium Scholar and intends on obtaining a master's degree in public health. As a Philadelphia native, Mr. Taylor plans on giving back to his city as a health care provider. He intends on matriculating into medical school after completing his masters in the fall of 2019 with hopes of obtaining an M.D./M.P.H. dual degree. Mr. Taylor has worked as a research assistant for a hospital-based violence intervention program in Philadelphia, Healing Hurt People. The program is designed to reduce recidivism among youth seen in emergency departments for violence-related injuries. During his time with the program, he was introduced to the importance of a trauma-informed approach for ending the cycle of violence. Mr. Taylor is interested in pursuing a career in emergency medicine. He desires to help combat health care issues affecting urban communities.

Robert Wardlow is currently a 6th-year M.D./Ph.D. candidate in the Medical Scientist Training Program at the Johns Hopkins University School of Medicine. His Ph.D. work, in the laboratory of Hal Dietz, entails studying the genetic underpinnings of hereditary aneurysm disorders such as Marfan syndrome. Mr. Wardlow grew up primarily in Cherry Hill, New Jersey, and graduated in 2012 from the University of Maryland, Baltimore County, with a B.S. in biochemistry and molecular biology.